I0135096

LIVES PARALLELED

Living in Shadows and Light

JESSICA GALLIGANI, C.HOM.

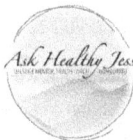

Ask Healthy Jess

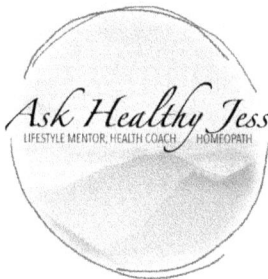

AskHealthyJess.com
ISBN 978-1-7348710-3-6
All rights reserved.
© 2020 Jessica Galligani

All rights reserved. No part of this publication may be reproduced, stored or transmitted in any form or by any means, electronic, mechanical, photocopying, recording, scanning, or otherwise without written permission from the publisher. It is illegal to copy this book, post it to a website, or distribute it by any other means without permission.

Jessica Galligani asserts the moral right to be identified as the author of this work.

Jessica Galligani has no responsibility for the persistence or accuracy of URLs for external or third-party Internet Websites referred to in this publication and does not guarantee that any content on such Websites is, or will remain, accurate or appropriate.

Dedication

This book evolved due to the many people who have influenced my life. I can't possibly list every single one of you, because the truth is, even strangers we encounter and words shared with a fleeting passersby can influence us at our very core. I would, however like to specifically thank those who are closest to me, and please know that if you are in my life, I value you as part of our journey, even if your name isn't listed here.

I want to thank my husband, David, for supporting every goal I have mustered up throughout the years. Without your encouragement and the many hours you have taken over the details of life in our busy home so I could submerge myself in writing, I couldn't have made this book a reality. You stood beside me every single step of the way while life unfolded before us, no matter how much it challenged us.

I would like to thank my beautiful boys, Grayson and Gavin, for giving me this purpose in life and for choosing us as your parents. You brought light and order to an otherwise senseless world. You inspire me to think out of the box and to right every wrong creatively and intentionally. I love you both with everything I am.

I want to thank my mother, sisters and brother for their roles in our journey, as well as the many other dear souls I have had the honor of knowing and loving who have aided in my growth and development: my sister-in-law Jenna, my friend Nicole, Miss Michele, who was Grayson's preschool Montessori teacher, and my very dear spiritual leaders and friends: Stephanie, Jill, Tami, and Leticia. I also want to thank Kaire for taking the time to provide valuable feedback when I was just starting this book, regurgitating some of the deepest memories of the last nine years of my life.

The beautiful people who helped me pull this project together as I stumbled through the steps of self-publishing are my editors Laura Hirsch and Sophie Elletson, cover designer Damon Freeman, and copywriter Bryan Cohen.

Writing a memoir spurs an invaluable piece of healing. I'm grateful for this opportunity to share our story with you. So thank you to YOU, the reader, for giving our story purpose.

Contents

Introduction

This is a narrative about how we navigated life with an Autism Spectrum Disorder (ASD) and Pediatric Autoimmune Neuropsychiatric Disorder Associated with Streptococcus (PANDAS) diagnosis. You can replace these conditions with any environmentally influenced illness, cognitive or degenerative disease like multiple sclerosis, dementia, allergies, arthritis, ADHD and the like. Although they may express themselves differently in each individual body, they are often rooted in the very same soil - over-toxification and under-methylation. Sherry Rogers, a doctor specializing in environmental medicine states,

> *"Toxicity is a one-way street leading to disease; the key to healing the impossible is to reverse the toxicity."*

What we have learned through our journey is that "toxicity" is not purely a physical phenomenon, although it does play an important role in the big picture. In susceptible people, we must consider the underlying terrain and how it evokes a result like dis-ease or disharmony in the body.

Many have been falsely led to believe that genetics alone are the cause. This theory is not only inaccurate, but it removes your power in the situation. If genetics alone was responsible for the majority of illnesses, recovery from them wouldn't be possible, yet I have personally known hundreds of people with stories like ours, ranging from previously non-verbal autism to wheelchair-bound multiple sclerosis. Genetic susceptibility does NOT have to result in illness, not even in old age. We must first believe in our power to avert the course we are on, only then are we open enough to seek answers to the puzzle before us.

The pages you are about to read are a raw account of the most important years of my life. My ultimate goal in writing this book is simply to encourage trust in your own intuitive gauge, igniting a sense of hope for your path to unfold before you, with beauty and enlightenment, that is only yours to experience. As you immerse yourself into our world on the following pages, allow your intuition to kick in and spark your own inspiration for healing.

Our son's recovery from ASD and PANDAS unveiled my own path. This journey is about these beautifully intertwined paths and how relying on one another for the direction of our evolution was the light at the end of the tunnel. I have discovered unmistakable purpose from the depths of our darkest days to the top of our most glorious moments as a family.

When asked if I would do it all over again, just the way it unfolded, I respond with a resounding yes! Would I have made it to this point if I chose another path? Well, I don't know, because I think I am always where I am supposed to be. Every step of the way, I learned something new. We needed the path we were on. We are who we are today *because* of the path we have traveled. We saw glimpses of who our children could be, and it drove us harder. We learned about anatomy and physiology *because* of the path we traveled. Our diets are healthy and our environment is cleaned up *because* of the research we did. We researched and experimented and we came to incredible conclusions due to the roads we traveled.

Most importantly, we met the people we needed to meet to find this path. It wasn't put in front of us sooner for very valid reasons, *we just weren't ready for it*! Every single day of our pasts have lead us to this very point in our lives. We wouldn't change a thing. Without the first IgG food sensitivity panel, we wouldn't have known to cut problematic foods which resulted in healthier eating habits for the whole family. Without the use of natural antimicrobials, we wouldn't have learned the signs of microbial overgrowth or how important it was to address the infections even if we would eventually change the way we handle them. Without learning about the Andy Cutler Chelation Protocol which involved low dose, oral supplementation to remove heavy metals from the body, we wouldn't have known that the toxicity of heavy metals are a problem in our world, which opened my awareness and spurred change towards a healthier lifestyle overall. Without the implementation of soil-based organisms, we wouldn't have dropped all of the antimicrobials we were using daily, proving that building up the gut terrain was more effective than tearing it down. Without the experience of Homotoxicology, a homeopathic method of opening the detox pathways, we wouldn't have eliminated dozens of supplements, and without homeopathy and energy healing, we wouldn't have the permanent healing we have experienced. Even camel's milk had its place on our healing path. Most importantly, I wouldn't have crossed paths with some of the most influential people in our lives.

As we make our choices, we are bringing all of who we are into that decision. We will make what we may later perceive as the wrong one, but is it really? Have you learned from making mistakes? What if we choose to see each "mistake" as the next step in our evolution rather than something that wasn't supposed to happen? Consider the conscious shift that will take place when we begin to welcome these lessons into our lives. This alone will change our trajectory.

Our jagged path to recovery is sprinkled with moments of clarity which came from what most people would call a "gut feeling" or what I like to refer to as "mother's intuition." I am not implying that you should do exactly what I did in order to find healing. Quite the contrary, I hope this book encourages you to unearth YOUR personal road to recovery.

Welcome to our long and winding path to recovery from Autism and PANDAS! Here you will see our lessons unravel into a beautiful recovery, full of light and hope for others making their way through this same confusing jungle.

Life is definitely what we make of it, don't underestimate the power of your journey. I'm sure my path is intersecting with yours for a very good reason.

Forward by Grayson

The child in this book *used* to have Autism. The child in this book *used* to have PANDAS. The child in this book is *healed* from those things today, and is proof that this stuff can be healed and prevented. Also, the child in this book is me (in case you couldn't tell).

I am proof that it is possible that you can heal these things. I am ALSO proof perfect people are real (just kidding (probably)). I don't really remember all that much that happened back when I was Autistic, just a little bit. I'm sure you don't remember your entire childhood either, so don't blame me. I do know that all that matters is what I am like now, and the journey we took to get here.

Everything we did to change my life was hard but worth it. Everything from getting rid of a lot (and I mean a LOT) of foods, like gluten, dairy, soy, and corn to name a few, to lowering screen time (that one was, and still is, hard) was tough at times, but you can get used to it.

As long as you follow the path we made for you, you can make it to where we are now (unless we keep progressing. We kind of had a few of years for a head start sooooooo… yeah.).

If your kid was how I used to be, don't you want to help them no matter how hard it is? If it were your parents, you would want them to do the same for you. Jessica, my mom, wrote this book so you can follow our journey. We beat down a path so you can follow, instead of having to beat one down yourself.

—Grayson (age 14), Jessica's Recovered Son

———

The cover photo was taken by me when Grayson was rounding the corner of recovery. The pride displayed for this piece of artwork is evident in his smile. It's an emotion that wasn't expressed for many years prior.

The artwork was entered into a cover page contest for a sustainability project that was due to be presented at schools across the Nation and we won! This image was the face of that sustainability project! We couldn't be more proud.

For us personally, this image represents so many things about our journey. It clearly aligns subtly with the Autism puzzle theme, but more importantly, it represents the global crisis we are facing with Autism and PANDAS, and many other chronic conditions. Equally however, it represents the spreading awareness and knowledge of holistic healing for chronic conditions like Autism and PANDAS which were once considered unchangeable. We hope to touch a lot of hearts across the globe with our message.

So eloquently put by Grayson's Grandma Galligani, "He's holding his future, his cure, his life in his hands!"

PART I

OUR STORY

AUTISM AND PANDAS WERE THE LESSONS, AN AWAKENING WAS THE RESULT

It's a new life!

LITERALLY AND FIGURATIVELY

"Loving a child doesn't mean giving in to all his whims; to love him is to bring out the best in him, to teach him to love what is difficult."

-Nadia Boulanger

AFTER THIRTEEN HOURS of intense labor, a new life enters our world on May 28, 2005 at 1:35pm. Grayson's beautiful little round face stares up at me, peacefully scanning me like he is reading my soul.

"Grayson," I say to myself as I hold him. I am still flabbergasted that he is here already. Nine months of preparation didn't prepare me for this moment, not one bit. It was even better than I had imagined, it was magical. Ready or not, here we go!

I AM the much older sister to my three siblings who ranged from nine to seventeen years younger than me. I spent many years co-parenting them with my single mother, yet this still feels so foreign to me. Holding and cuddling him came natural, but the figurative weight on my shoulders, ouch! He's ours and ours alone, he relies completely on us for survival, happiness, and guidance. Much of what he is going to experience hinges on us as his parents. Gulp. No pressure though!

At first, it felt like we were playing house. Let's take him for a walk, dress him up, take his picture, he loves when you hold him like this, and so on. But those grueling nights when he slept for a whole hour at a time told me otherwise. We weren't playing, this was our reality! And the days he spent wailing for various reasons unknown to us at the time, reminded us that his health and happiness were ours to unravel...and it felt like we were failing miserably! Little did we know, this blessed little soul entered our world ready to teach us much of what we would eventually value beyond life itself.

THE FIRST YEAR of Grayson's life was filled with contradictory emotions for us as parents. His first everything was beautiful to experience, but all rolled up with these joyous experiences were the hovering shadows of something confusing. Grayson was an intense baby right from day one. He was born with spunk. Immediately following his birth, he lifted his upper body off the table with incredible strength, he also frequently pulled away from our cuddles with that same strength. He was never happy sitting still. I had an inkling he would be active, just based on his activity levels during my pregnancy, but after his birth, it was obvious that he was bright and alert, and also extremely fidgety. It was actually hard to hold him as an infant, it was as if merely touching him was so disturbing to his senses that he couldn't sit still. We used to joke that he was ready to run before he could even hold himself upright and his strength was astonishing, his legs could hold his full body weight even as a newborn.

He was also very unique in many other ways, he was an incredibly quick learner, he was SO smart it was mind-blowing, but he was also easily startled by any sudden movements toys would make, he had to be swaddled until after he grew out of the swaddles and I had to cut the bottom open so he could still use them, he began rocking incessantly within his first year of life, he sucked his fingers until they bled and he couldn't tolerate dirty hands as he was learning to eat table food. The response to these upsets in his little life was strong enough to set off warning bells for me. Life as a baby shouldn't be stressful. Later, I would learn that my own stress-vibes about his emotional triggers, would further fuel his out of proportion responses.

My reality

OUR WORLD IS FLIPPED UPSIDE DOWN, THIS DOESN'T FEEL NORMAL

"I've got the key to my castle in the air, but whether I can unlock the door remains to be seen."

-Louisa May Alcott

"WHY WON'T HE NURSE??" I cried, and threw my head back in sync with my hungry newborn who was arching and writhing in my exhausted arms. He clearly wasn't happy and I didn't know what to do, so I did what everyone around me kept telling me to do: I stuck a bottle of formula in his mouth before he reached three months old...silence!! He's happy!! But I wasn't happy, it didn't feel right. What was in these formula powders anyway? I'll check later, I needed sleep and peace so desperately, and so did he, I just went with it. This was one of the many times I would stuff down my mama gut-feeling.

After all, thousands of other babies survived on formula, didn't they? It never occurred to me that the following months of doctor-diagnosed colic were directly related to the very formula that filled his hungry little tummy.

"WHY WON'T HE SLEEP??" came the next exasperated question out of my wearied mouth. I expected to lose sleep with a newborn, but at almost six months old, we were still struggling horribly with sleep. We had not enjoyed even a partial night's sleep since the day we brought him home. He would grumble and wrestle and toss and turn, eventually working himself up to an all-out wail every 45 minutes to an hour. Hungry? No, he just ate and turned away from his bottle. Wet? Nope, not that either. Try some cuddles...he pushed away. In hindsight, he was probably terribly uncomfortable because his gut flora was imbalanced and he was rejecting cow dairy, which we would later learn was a significant problem for him. If I had known then what I know now about the importance of beneficial bacteria, I might have known to give him a probiotic and alter my diet, but as a new mom with no experience in this, I was using my good old standby, "What to Expect" books. They don't explain that an infant develops his/her gut flora from mom during childbirth, nor does it explain how vital these beneficial bacteria are in the role of health and wellness. A large number of neurotransmitters are found in the gut, where eighty percent of our immune system is located. In fact, roughly ninety-five percent of serotonin is produced in the gut, so it goes without saying that anything which has an impact on our intestines, has an equal impact on our neurology. Grayson's physical struggles were flying under my radar, because I was uneducated at the time.

I had to go to sleep beside him at 7pm in order to achieve a full 4 hours of continuous sleep, because beyond that, he was up hourly, sometimes more often! Thankfully, "The Baby Whisperer's" gentle sleep training techniques came to the rescue, and with very diligent consistency, we managed to squeak more sleep out of him at six months old, although it still wasn't great. I was happy though, well happier anyway. Was he?

. . .

WHEN GRAYSON WAS ONLY a few months old, I walked into his room to check on him napping, one of my many intuitive hits about his health, and instead of glancing in to find a peacefully sleeping baby, I witnessed the kind of stillness that can rip out a parent's heart. I watched for that relieving raise of the chest to signify a breath, and none came. I felt as though the wind had been knocked out of me, which appeared to be how he felt too. I scooped him up hastily, with every intent of waking him and was grateful when he woke startled and deeply gasped back to breathing normally. Had I imagined it? It all happened so quickly. No…a mother knows. I was still numb, it felt as though every blood cell instantly rushed to my limbs. My heart fluttered with pain while my head felt like it might float away. I was swarmed with fears, shaking from head to toe.

Of course, I did what any concerned parent would do and brought him to his pediatrician, where they promptly prescribed an at-home sleep apnea machine which would not only sound an alarm when he stopped breathing, but it would digitally track his breathing for us on a memory card. I had a love-hate relationship with that thing. It was an incredibly annoying contraption, because he had to be wired in multiple locations all over his body. Considering he required tight swaddling in order to sleep, it certainly made midnight feedings and diaper changes gripping with action…don't accidentally pull at a cord, it was like stepping on a mine!! The blaring alarm would pierce the silent nighttime air like a siren on a firehouse. We were equally grateful for the deafening alarm though, because with it brought security. We knew without a doubt, we wouldn't miss a beat if Grayson were to stop breathing. Neither would our neighbors, I bet!

We experienced the alarm a handful of times in those grueling weeks and although he did experience a few apnea episodes, they weren't considered troubling to doctors. At least by following the trends of his sleeping routines, we received some reassurance, but that little twinge of mama intuition was poking at me, reminding me that something more was at play here. More intuition stuffing.

It didn't dawn on us until much later, and many books later, that we could be dealing with vaccine damage. Knowing how many vaccinations are given in those first few months, there would be no way to know one way or the other if they were somehow at play here. We didn't have the knowledge to question vaccinations at the time, but this wouldn't be the last time something troubled us about Grayson's health.

As FIRST TIME PARENTS, my husband David and I remained excited and enthusiastic. We rejoiced in seeing life through our little one's eyes, the newness of life itself, things we had previously taken for granted. The smell of a flower, the excitement of flashing lights and even the unique and dependent affection for a cuddly "lovey." So why the undertone of stress? We had aspirations of fairytale happiness for our first born, but instead we felt distressed frequently. I can't lie, it was downright disappointing at times. The first experience of grass on his bare feet and he curled hesitantly and painfully away, he avoided barefoot grass even though we regularly spent hours outside barefoot, we had a pool after all! Yet still, we had hope and we continued to enjoy every budding moment with him. Such confusing moments woven throughout a time that was also teaming with beauty and bliss.

That first year was a whirlwind! I cried a lot of tears. I didn't realize how many more tears would be shed in the years to come. After Grayson's twelve-month vaccinations, we were really put to the test. I had taken him to visit my mother in Connecticut shortly after he was vaccinated with the MMR, Prevnar and Polio. Early in our trip, I noticed he was incredibly fussy and had developed visibly large, swollen glands, one on the side of his neck (cervical) and one to the side of his groin (inguinal). This was only the beginning of a slew of symptoms that followed for an entire month, back to back! Immediately following the swollen glands, while we were still away from home, he developed a high fever and full body rashes that resembled Rubella which moved all over his body right before my eyes. These weren't like raised hives, they were flat and lacy, and they were mobile! I'd never seen anything like it. He also developed large weeping bumps on his behind which resembled blisters that came and went over a period of days. He was miserable, lethargic and fussy, and I was terrified as a result.

I called our pediatrician who told us it was likely a virus. During this call, I remembered noticing a red circle on the top of his very fair head, just before our trip. Could it be Lyme Disease? I would normally be fine with accepting this as a virus, but something wasn't sitting right, my gut was telling me something wasn't right and that it wasn't a virus, it was too bizarre. This is when we began dabbling in homeopathy for Grayson. We grabbed some remedies for vaccine reactions down at the local health food store out of sheer desperation. His rashes subsided, but the fever raged on and he was so visibly uncomfortable.

As soon as we returned home, we took him to the doctor and by then, he had accumulated a few more symptoms which were also brushed off with their cavalier lack of attention. One of his eyelids swelled up for a few days and shortly afterwards he couldn't bend the same knee where the vaccine was given in his thigh. Thankfully, that didn't last very long. He ended the spree of symptoms with hives which the doctor thought was from a food he had eaten, something he had eaten many times before and had gone on to eat since then (with no hives). Then he got a good old fashioned ear infection. He had numerous ear infections in his first year of life starting at only weeks old, so we were not strangers to the course of antibiotics that would follow. At the time, I didn't know to question repeated courses of antibiotics, I was a diligent patient following doctor's orders. Meanwhile, the swollen glands remained...for six years!

The troublesome number of tests he was put through was enough to drive a sensitive parent crazy, but we were driven by the need for answers. I couldn't stand a single additional blood draw for my little guy who was already terrified just walking through the front door of our pediatrician's office at this point. He literally began crying and clawing at me at the sight of this door, I can't even imagine the trauma it caused him.

He was tested for inflammatory autoimmune diseases like Lupus and Arthritis, as well as Lyme disease, which was negative (if only I knew then what I know now about Lyme testing accuracy). They ran a host of other labs, including things that would rule out Leukemia. The only positive finding was that he was experiencing "inflammation" suggested by a high Sed Rate, or erythrocyte sedimentation rate (ESR). An inflammatory marker like the Sed Rate is very generic and doesn't provide information about where the inflammation is or what caused it, so the only thing we knew is that our baby was suffering with some form of systemic inflammation. When we asked the doctor what it meant, it was shrugged off with a nondescript explanation of inflammation.

I still didn't know if this was truly a vaccine reaction or if the vaccines just stressed his immune system enough to activate potential congenital Lyme disease or a latent virus. Only bio-resonance testing has confirmed Lyme disease in our family, but we also never tried testing with a more reputable lab like Igenex. Either way, this was ultimately the reason we finally began questioning vaccinations. We weren't yet convinced that we needed to stop them entirely so we continued to allow a chosen few, one at a time, and even the pediatrician agreed - no live viruses. In due diligence, we researched more and eventually stopped all together.

My strength pulled me through all the testing, and the dreaded anticipation of lab results, one after another, but when we reached the calm (and all labs were clear, not perfect, but nothing telling) I hit an all-time low. It had taken all I had to maintain composure through the ups and downs. I had feared the worst, Leukemia. You would think it would be good news, to have nothing glaring in all the testing that was done, but all it did was serve to drive my burning fears further into my soul, because something still wasn't right. I was haunted by the events and convinced that something big was looming, it just wasn't showing up on labs. I was quickly losing faith in the medical field. They had no answers, and of course, our speculation that this was in direct relation to his recent slew of vaccines was brushed under the rug. It went on record as "Mom worried, maybe from shots." His glands were still permanently swollen and he was growing increasingly sensitive to external stimuli. I just couldn't let it go, thoughts spiraled around in my head constantly and I couldn't control them anymore. The little sleep I was getting was fractured and filled with nightmares about what might be impending.

I no longer wanted to go anywhere or do anything, simply taking a shower was even beginning to feel like a chore. It was as if the life had been sucked out of my body, I was a shell of a person. It took everything I had just to feed Grayson, let alone myself, and I knew that somehow I needed to function better for my family. At my husband's (strong) recommendation, I began seeing someone for therapy and I hesitantly began taking an antidepressant.

DAVE HAD ALWAYS BEEN an easy going partner in our relationship. When I met him and his soft blue eyes greeted mine, I instantly felt a jab at my heart. I knew he was the one who could hold onto my heart forever. I can't even tell you how I knew this, I just did. From that moment forward, he was by my side, an enthusiastic and active participant, but very gentle in his persuasion. He gracefully balanced my somewhat hardened personality. It was rare for him to use decisive words, because in his mind, everything really was always going to be "just fine."

This time however, I can recall the anxiety in his body and voice like it was yesterday. This was putting him way outside of his comfort zone and he was serious when he said to me, "Jessica, I think it might be worth going to see someone, this isn't healthy for you, or Grayson. He needs you." I knew he was right and I hated that he was right! I felt broken and torn, like a tattered old rag. The past six weeks had drained me of all the will I had left. The thought that I was letting my family down added to the pressure I put on myself. I am normally a tough cookie, my childhood required me to mature before most even knew what the word meant, but this was uncharted territory and I agreed with my husband, I needed profes-sional help. We both knew that things couldn't go on this way. I caved, and I leaned on my reliable husband for support.

I was officially diagnosed as depressed. No surprise there! I used medication only long enough (and at a fraction of an adult dose) to return to my rational self. Besides, it was nice to enjoy showers again! I'm sure Dave would agree. I was ultimately able to eliminate the medication with the assistance of a homeopath in India. She was truly my light at the end of what felt like a long and terrifying, dark tunnel. She also served to turn me on to homeopathy as a superior form of medicine. My personal experience with home-opathy made me a believer. My remedy was powerful enough to replace Prozac. If anxiety or fearful thoughts crept in, a few of those magical little white pellets was all it took for me to bounce back. Before long, I didn't even need them at all.

She tried to find effective remedies for Grayson's vaccine reac-tions, unfortunately, with little success. I would later learn about a phenomenon known in homeopathy as a "maintaining cause" or "the obstacle to the cure" which is an ongoing event that prevents remedies from working. It was likely that his lack of response to treatment was due to various maintaining causes that blocked healing for him. I maintained my faith in homeopathy since it was working so incredibly well for me, but the costs were restrictive and the results weren't enough to remain with her any longer for Grayson. If there was one thing in my past that I regret, it's not trying another homeopath at this time, but it wasn't meant to be. I had many lessons to learn still.

3

Autism?!

"*You will face your greatest opposition when you are closest to your biggest miracle.*"

-Shanon L. Alder

NOT LONG AFTER Grayson's second birthday, we were delighted to learn that I was pregnant with our second son. A brother for Grayson was the plan, but I would soon learn that the task of juggling an infant along with what was next on our list of responsibilities, would prove to test our endurance.

We were still trying to rationalize the intense reactions Grayson was having to sensory stimuli. The wind was too painful, the sun was too hot, his food was either too hot or cold, his hands couldn't be dirty, socks and shoes were always too tight or too loose, he covered his ears with his hands and screamed in response to loud sounds. He literally scaled my husband's 6'1" body when a motorcycle drove through the neighborhood and he punched me in the face for flushing a public toilet. He had a heck of a right hook!

We also noticed that he was beginning to flap his hands wildly when he was excited in any way, positively or negatively, and he had developed a new movement we coined as "swatting." It looked as though he had flies zipping around his head, he would swat around his ears over and over again, every few seconds. We later learned that this was the start of his array of tics associated with PANDAS. You will learn more about our growing awareness of PANDAS as it unfolds along our journey, which is peppered with events as we experienced them. We also noticed he was unnaturally fascinated by ceiling fans. He would stare at them for great lengths of time, as if they hypnotized him.

The pile-up of these odd events had me looking for more answers. Doctors felt his eye contact was "normal" and he was "so smart," there was nothing to worry about. By two, he knew his numbers, shapes, colors and alphabet including many of their phonetic sounds, but this didn't help comfort me regarding his shifting and unsettling behaviors. A mother knows her child, she knows when something doesn't feel right, but again, I was stuffing my intuition to appease everyone around me who thought I was reading into things. "Don't look for something that isn't there," "Let's give it some time, I bet he will grow out of these things," "He's too young to tell," were among the many things I heard from the people around me. Meanwhile, I felt like I was losing precious time trying to figure out why he was regressing instead of developing appropriately. I was still very unsettled and by now, as you can imagine, I was educating myself on Google University at great lengths. I began reading a book called "The Highly Sensitive Child." I was grasping at anything in an attempt to ease the discomfort that was rising in the pit of my stomach.

And then it happened. It was bound to happen with my eternal quest for information...I came across the "red flags" for Autism one night during my endless hours of research.

Silence

Only the sound of the whirring computer fan kicking on could be heard as I sat motionless, staring at the screen in front of me. Words on the screen, staring back at me staring at them. Autism, it instantly cuts like a knife through the hopes and dreams a parent has for her child. Numb was to become my new norm. I was instantly fear-stricken, the kind of fear associated with instant full-body sweat. I had never handled the unknown well, and this was no exception. Questions swirled in my head as the growing pit in my stomach exploded with enough force to make me want to vomit.

What did this mean? Could my child actually be on this "spectrum" I was reading about? And if he was, what next? I had only encountered one other child with Autism and she couldn't speak. I quickly composed myself and tried to reassure myself. He didn't have *all* the symptoms and they often came and went. I didn't want to believe it, but the fiery crater in my stomach told me I had found exactly what I was looking for.

As if this wasn't enough, we were also in the midst of a move to a new home, our dream home. This move was supposed to cradle us with warm feelings and set the stage for new and lofty family dreams. Instead, I was in great turmoil and didn't know where to turn for answers about my brewing concerns, and the move only added to my stress.

At this point, symptoms began to arrive faster than I could keep up with. Grayson's sensory-seeking behavior was off the charts. He would throw himself around our house like a rag doll, bumping and crashing into everything around him, including people. That didn't go over well on play dates! It wasn't like he was out of control or couldn't walk normally, he clearly just chose not to. Jumping was his form of transportation. Crashing wasn't limited to furniture, he crashed into us, the floor, toys! He was even cramming his hands deeply between the cushions of the couch for that same sort of sensory input, it gave him the sensation of pressure on his joints.

He began new routine habits, like tracing our cabinet drawers/doors with his fingers and he wouldn't tolerate interruption until he completed the one he was on. Once he had begun tracing a cabinet, his thoughts couldn't be interrupted until the task was completed. There was an intense hyper-focus about it which felt like it was anxiety-driven. We didn't recognize it at the time, but this was the start of his obsessive compulsive disorder (OCD) symptoms. Transitions from one activity to another became a nightmare and he even began to lose eye contact at times. I knew I had to do something when his unnecessary routines became so rigid that they were disruptive to life in our home. Leaving the house became more and more laborious, to the point where we began isolating ourselves from the outside world and everyone in it.

ONE EXAMPLE of how our lives were impacted by things that most people don't even take notice of, involves wrinkles in sheets. When he was going to sleep, wrinkles in his bedding caused out of control tantrums that prevented sleep for hours. And the pillow, oh gosh, the pillow couldn't be off center between the two sides of his bed. Dave handled the nighttime routine with him, and thankfully he had so much more patience than I did, maybe because he was able to decompress at work while I was fully submerged in this twenty four hours a day. He would cheerfully tuck Grayson in, while reassuring him that everything would be ok, smoothing out the wrinkles and centering the pillow for him, then RE-smoothing out wrinkles that formed as he rose from the bed, just to be called back in with wails and fits of fury, "I can't sleeeeep!!," as he angrily and frantically smoothed and pressed each little wrinkle, then shifted his pillow from side to side. To our dismay, there was very little we could do to ease his growing frenzy once it started.

One unforgettable night I was home alone with both boys while Dave was traveling for business. Grayson had come out of his room furious about his sheets, and when he was upset to this point, he would sweat and get very itchy, which added to his increasing irritability. The air was taught with friction. I began by trying to comfort and distract him, thinking that maybe if I could just hug him until he calmed, he might be able to fall asleep.

Gently I consoled him, "Shhhhhh, it's ok Grayson, shhhhhh, why don't you come sit with me."

With violent outrage he pushed and fought and in a low guttural voice, he snarled at me, "Let GO of me RIGHT NOOOOW! LET GO OF MEEEE! DON'T TOUCH ME!" In defeat, I let go, sat back and sobbed into my hands. I wanted to help my little boy, but he wasn't even capable of finding refuge in the cradles of his mother's arms.

We eventually learned that by tucking the blankets in VERY tightly under either side of the mattress, wrinkles are almost nonexistent, and the added bonus of the sensory input of a taught blanket offered additional comfort, but the pillow was still a problem. We were grateful for the little things. Living on eggshells taught us to celebrate every little creative solution that brought momentary peace into our lives. We lived for the moments Grayson smiled, because they were fleeting, as his anger appeared to be looming more often.

Eating three meals a day came with the fear of more outbursts, because Grayson's chair HAD to be the same exact distance from the legs of the table on both sides, I swear, to the millimeter!! He would abruptly yank his screeching chair back and forth and back and forth, over and over, crying tears of defeat when it wasn't just right. With each angry shove of the chair, he would push it further away from his desired destination, his outrage causing him to push harder and harder, losing sight of his purpose in the first place, until he was wrapped up in a fit of tears and angst. To make matters worse, my inability to comfort him. He would finally get settled just long enough for his fork to fall off of his plate and cause him to fall apart yet again. Everyday tasks were resulting in this sort of response. All. Day. Long. What little resolve I had was dwindling.

**To SEE our list of symptoms, go to Chapter 7 in PART II - THE RESOURCE GUIDE.

4

Turning point

HOW DIETARY INTERVENTION SPARKS
NEW HOPE

"Thou canst not travel on the path before thou hast become the path itself."

-H.P. Blavatsky

I BELIEVE that experiences enter our lives with purpose and in a very timely manner. If we are open to these messages and we trust our instincts about them, we will find ourselves on the path which suits us best. We had been feverishly searching for answers when a business reward trip brought Dave and I to Arizona for a week. A much needed break before the new baby was due to arrive! We would learn about one huge piece of our puzzle in Arizona. It would trigger the first of many changes. I credit this experience with giving me the strength I needed to find real answers.

While we were soaking up the rays by the pool at the resort one sunny day in Arizona, a fellow salesperson in the company was sitting at the edge of the pool chatting with a few others about her daughter, who had recently been diagnosed with Asperger's syndrome. I was mysteriously drawn to her conversation, as if being pushed to listen to her. I tuned into her conversation and my ears perked up, because I heard her describing some of her daughter's behaviors from pre-diagnosis. She was explaining how simply changing her diet had eliminated a good portion of her symptoms. I made my way over to her side of the pool and took a dip while listening for an opening where I could comfortably make myself part of the conversation. As if she sensed my earnest interest, her eyes met mine, she smiled, she knew.

What I learned that day catapulted me into what would result in years upon years of research. It started that very day when I returned to our hotel room to Google the gluten-free, casein-free diet. I was hungry for information. It offered hope! It also confirmed what I thought we were dealing with, Grayson likely had some form of Autism Spectrum Disorder (ASD). Oddly though, by reading more about it, I was becoming less frightened of it. I was feeling empowered by information. I read books and researched online for literally 6-8 hours almost daily for many of the next 5 years.

Upon returning home, we began experimenting with his diet by removing gluten and casein (dairy protein). Interestingly, it was when we removed these foods that we realized exactly how much he had been self-limiting to gluten and casein containing foods! A two-year-old shouldn't be drinking milk four times a day still! This self-limiting of problematic foods is one of the tell-tale signs that a child is sensitive to them, which of course, I learned in one of my endless reading spurts. When we took them out, we felt like we were left with nothing to feed him. If only we knew how much more we would eventually have to limit his diet in the future, this might have felt like a piece of cake!! Hindsight is 20/20! We saw some improvements which were noticeable, but nothing earth shattering. His behavior was still a wild roller coaster ride most days.

5

Change is in the air

EVEN THE OVER-STIMULATION OF TOO MUCH EXCITEMENT CAN TAKE ITS TOLL

"*T*here is nothing permanent except change."

-Heraclitus

IT IS POSSIBLE for too much of a good thing to create imbalance. We were on the cusp of so much change, all great changes by our standards, but was it too much too fast?

On the afternoon of June 25, 2008, Grayson's baby brother Gavin entered our lives fast and furiously. I had a quick and easy labor and delivery, although he did encounter a few glitches along the way. My placenta had ruptured during labor and the cord was prolapsed for a short period during delivery so there was concern of reduced oxygen. He was brought to the NICU for a few hours of monitoring, but joined us in my room before the next morning. His timely arrival was a welcome change to our stressed routines. He reminded us that there was so much more to our lives than the narrow-minded focus fear had reduced us to lately. We were ready to grace our new little boy with love and affection. He added so much joy and light to our family. Gavin was a champ at nursing and such a cuddly little mama's boy. I reveled in his desire for touch and the endearing way he watched me, as I watched him nursing. Grayson took his arrival very well, almost too well.....he was gentle with his baby brother, although he didn't show much interest either. He seemed indifferent and just went about his day playing, without paying much attention to the changes going on around him.

IN JUST UNDER A YEAR, we had uprooted our home and moved, had a new baby and put Grayson in preschool. I realize now, this was a lot of stress for a three-year-old to manage, and it showed. He was already struggling before we moved, and with the added life changes, he too was changing rapidly before our eyes. We had entered him into a very small (six kids per classroom), peaceful Montessori preschool for three half-days per week. We knew he was sensitive to extra stimuli, yet he craved social interaction. He was such a fast learner that we wanted him to be in an environment that would welcome his advanced curiosity. By the time he was three, he was already teaching himself to read, by three and a half, he had learned where just about every country in the world was. His teacher even called him a "geographical genius." He was like a little sponge sopping up everything he was surrounded by!

Surprisingly though, shortly after starting school, things took a serious turn for the worse. His behavior was radically different suddenly. He loved school, he looked forward to every day there, and was clearly learning, but why wasn't his behavior lining up with his feelings? I began to dread picking him up from school, because each day there was a new "behavior" to discuss. I felt like I was driving straight to the principal's office each day. I was such a goody two shoes growing up, and this was so against every cell in my body. I felt like a failure as a mom. How had I failed him?

One particular afternoon, as usual, the owner of the school came out to greet me, smiling in her apologetic way. A pang of nervousness hit as I felt the familiar sympathy that came with "the look." I know it was painful for her too. She was a sweet, soft-spoken and gentle mother of two herself. She always put on a smile and she spoke slowly and calmly, as if that would change the stress-charged stories she was obligated to report to me from his mornings in her care. As our eyes met, she smiled bigger briefly before painfully explaining that Grayson had taken his arm and swiped it clear across their dry erase calendar, erasing multiple days at once. He laughed through it all, then proceeded to strip his pants down to his ankles and roll around on the floor, laughing as if he were on a hysterical high. His behavior had become unmanageable at home these days, but this even surprised me! I was appalled. Was this Autism? On this day, his teacher, who was also the owner of the school, suggested that maybe "Montessori wasn't for him." No, no, no….I vehemently disagreed! This was the ONLY school for him. He would never thrive in the hustle and bustle of a public classroom where thirty children shared one teacher and chaos was the norm. In a shared moment of silence my eyes pleaded with her to give us time. She nodded as she glanced at the ground, she knew I was right. We were working on finding answers. I just needed time. We could handle this, we would have to handle this, for him. As if attempting to encourage herself, she hesitantly agreed that we would work on it together. She couldn't give up on us, and I greedily played on those emotions. She was vested in him and I remain grateful for her dedicated involvement in his early education experiences.

At home, things were still just as confusing. The icing on the cake for me was the incessant act of lining up cars. Rows and rows of cars that he didn't play with, he just lined them up perfectly, all over the house. And God forbid if we touch one or move something out of place, he would have a fit. We couldn't sit on our couches without accidentally sending the cars sliding this way and that way, instigating a new tantrum. I also noticed Grayson's self-esteem was plummeting. We were always so proud of his accomplishments and we encouraged him to try again when he didn't succeed the first time. His three short years of life were full of daily praise. Why was he so down on himself? Frequent words out of his mouth were, "I can't do it!" It was like he was in a toddler depression!

My heart was breaking for him, I didn't know what I could do to help him feel better and find peace. I finally broke down and made an appointment with a therapist to have him evaluated. He was already too old for early intervention who placed the cutoff for Sensory Processing Disorder therapy at three years old. I had been taking Gavin to physical therapy for Torticollis and during one of Gavin's sessions, the owner of the practice commented on Grayson's low muscle tone, another classic Autism sign, along with the sensory dysfunction, the lining up of cars, the hand flapping, the ceiling fan obsession, the swatting, the rigidity, the reduced eye contact, the compulsions and the out of proportion tantrums.

Doctors still weren't concerned, because he was so bright and charming. And he was, he was a very charming child. He wins everyone over with his high energy, charisma and his engaging smile, but like the car that doesn't act up when you take it to the mechanic, he was always on his best when he was on display for the doctors. He was capable of controlling himself in new situations. His inconsistencies had Dave believing we couldn't possibly be dealing with Autism. Having this assessment was an important first step in supporting what I knew I was seeing. I needed a professional on board. I couldn't fight this alone, not yet anyway.

The evaluation confirmed my suspicions. He had Sensory and Auditory Processing Disorder (SPD). It was on paper. NOW people were beginning to pay attention.

Sensory and Auditory Processing Disorder exists when sensory signals don't get organized appropriately within the nervous system. Rather than organizing the sensory signals appropriately, someone with SPD detects the information, but the signals get mixed up in the brain resulting in an unusual response to the sensory input. This disorder was contributing to Grayson's symptoms of being easily distracted and unusually upset by loud noises, difficulty following direction, comprehending abstract information, crashing into every-thing and anything, his repulsion to touch and cuddling, yet needing bear hugs, food texture aversions, his dissatisfaction with dirty hands, meltdowns in public places, and even his inability to calm down enough to fall asleep. Here we were, using a label, but unfortunately, sometimes a label is what is needed to set things in motion. In motion, we were.

6

The fork in the road

WHERE TRADITIONAL MODALITIES AND
ALTERNATIVE HEALING COLLIDE

"No problem can be solved from the same level of consciousness that created it."

-Albert Einstein

WITH THE SUGGESTION of occupational therapy multiple times per week, it was time to decide on a direction for treatment. Historically, treatment of Sensory Processing Disorder has been Occupational Therapy. This is the only treatment recognized by conventional medicine, as well as insurance companies. I just wasn't feeling it, after everything I had read about Biomedicine.

PER THE MERRIAM-WEBSTER DICTIONARY, Biomedicine is

"medicine based on the application of the principles of the natural sciences and especially biology and biochemistry; also: a branch of medical science concerned especially with the capacity of human beings to survive and function

in abnormally stressful environments and with the protective modification of such environments."

I understand the idea behind therapy, but the way my mind works is to go right to the cause. SPD was a symptom of the cause. Doing therapy when the cause isn't addressed felt like slapping a Bandaid on the boo-boo with dirt still on the wound. Why were his fine motor skills delayed, why couldn't he pinpoint individual sounds in a group of sounds, why couldn't he use both feet when descending on the stairs or zip his coat without looking?

In my research, I was finding many connections between SPD and food sensitivities, as well as yeast/candida overgrowth, all of which fit under the umbrella of Autism. I immersed myself in groups of parents with kids on the spectrum and began networking in Autism communities. It was almost unanimous, they eliminated problematic foods (not just gluten and casein, but many more) and when they treated the yeast overgrowth, the SPD "symptoms" ceased to exist. Therapy-shmerapy, I was going for gold! If we could eliminate the problem at the root, the situation requiring therapy would correct itself. I immediately stocked up on some of the recommended natural anti-microbial supplies and made an appointment with Grayson's doctor. We had been taking him to a holistic doctor who called himself a DAN! doctor and ironically, I didn't even know what that stood for when we chose to use him. DAN! stands for "Defeat Autism Now." Huh…funny how the Universe works. This is right where we were meant to be.

One of the first tests we were advised to consider is called an IgG food panel. IgG stands for Immunoglobulin G, which is the main antibody isotope in the blood that controls infection by binding to undesirable pathogens. When these immunoglobulins are elevated, it is typically an indication of infection. The IgG food panel is a much more precise test than the IgG blood level test which just looks at the general IgG level in the body and wouldn't tell you more explicitly why they are elevated. The IgG food panel determines an inappropriate immunoglobulin response to specific foods in the blood. For this sort of immune response to happen, the perfect storm must be present.

When a person has leaky gut, also known as intestinal permeability, the intestines lose their ability to effectively filter substances. The result of a "leaky" intestinal wall is the penetration of undigested food particles (among other things) into the blood stream. So, now you know technically what is occurring in simplified terms, let me paint a picture for you to establish a clear understanding of what was going on.

First, let's imagine the IgG guys as armored antibodies, they are always armed and ready to fight. As described above, these are the same guys that come out to play when you encounter an illness, like the chickenpox. The first time they encounter the foreign invader, they develop memory of the invader, the next time they will fight to the familiar invader's demise. Now, let's imagine a few innocent food particles taking a wrong turn and ending up in the bloodstream, because there are too many openings in that pesky intestinal wall. Large, undigested food particles don't belong in the blood stream so the IgG warriors go on high alert. They develop memory to these intruders the first time they are encountered. So guess what happens when these same foods continue to enter the bloodstream? You've got it, the IgG antibodies rise to the occasion (because it's their job and you want them doing their job, right?). Now what you have is a battle ground in the body with a constant attempt to fight off something as innocent as food. They don't discern between healthy foods and unhealthy foods, they just fight anything that inappropriately ends up in the blood stream. Not only is this a losing battle as long as the foods are consumed, but it means that the host (the person with leaky gut) feels pretty awful when this is going on.

Think about how you feel when your body is fighting an infection, you are drained, grumpy, tired, impatient, you have brain fog and other unsavory symptoms. So a person with leaky gut, who continues to eat the foods that his or her body is trying to "fight" off, generally isn't feeling 100%. An inflammatory cycle begins as the food particles are fought day after day. This is how chronic autoimmunity begins. Human tissue becomes collateral damage during this process, escalating things into what is referred to as an autoimmune response due to the sheer repetitive nature of the daily battles.

For your children, this is going to result in a display of ailments that can vary, such as: mood swings causing negative behaviors, sleep disturbances, crankiness, fatigue, headaches or migraines, poor immunity, brain fog, lack of concentration and many other potential manifestations of illness. Leaky gut can trigger or flare other disorders like celiac disease, asthma, IBS, ADD, ADHD, rheumatoid arthritis, Crohn's disease, Vitiligo and other autoimmune diseases. The sheer number of children being medicated for these exact symptoms is astounding, and growing. Learning disorders can be the result of sensitivities. Would you be able to study for an exam with a pending cold? No, you would probably rather lay in bed or sit in front of the TV, where the furthest thing from your mind would be mental activity.

Only recently, in 2019 a paper published in *"Annals of Neurology"* reported the presence of cellular features consistent with an immune response targeting specialized brain cells in more than two-thirds of Autistic brains analyzed postmortem.[1][2]

WITH THE RESULTS of Grayson's IgG food panel showing 23, yes that was TWENTY THREE foods that we had to remove from his diet, my first blog was born, *"You are what you eat!"* Many of the day-to-day details I decided not to bore you with in this book were written into my blog. On December 3, 2008, I posted my first entry.

Reality check

You are what you eat....This statement could never be more true in our house! I have always been into eating healthy and living healthy, but having a son newly diagnosed with several food allergies adds new meaning to that theory!!

Our adventure began with a diagnosis of SPD (sensory processing disorder). His sensory seeking behaviors, tantrums and low self-esteem was becoming increasingly more disturbing and when the behaviors began to effect life around our household, we knew we needed professional help. So in addition to seeking help for the SPD, we saw a wonderful holistic doctor who pointed us in the right direction. I also read a TON of great books addressing behavioral issues, SPD and even diet. I knew that there was a possibility that something he was eating could be effecting him so with the combination of therapy and diet intervention, I thought we could figure things out. And boy, I couldn't be more right!!

Fast forward to the current status of our household....a three year old who is always sweet to his baby brother, who has impeccable manners, is empathetic, smart beyond his years, glows with happiness and pride!

So what did we do differently you ask? We REMOVED allergenic foods that came up on an IgG blood test. Is it easy, heck no!! But it turns our child into the person he used to be, and I will do anything to keep him happy and healthy including baking, re-baking and baking again when the recipes turn out awful!! So if you thought meals in your house were challenging, try working without wheat, milk, eggs, rice, potatoes, kidney and pinto beans, coconut, cheese, asparagus, all citrus, pumpkin, olive (yes that includes the oil), canola oil, sesame....ugh!! There is at least one of these ingredients in just about everything! Not to mention the HIDDEN ingredients associated with wheat and milk. I have become a scientist, a chemist, a doctor and oddly enough, a chef! I HATE baking!! Luckily he can eat corn, because it seems like everything he DOES eat is from corn, corn chips, corn pasta, corn cereal, corn corn corn. [we eventually discovered that corn was a problem and lost this food too] *Another great replacement for us has been a grain called quinoa (pronounced KEEN wah), which is actually not really a grain at all, it's the seed of a fruit and contains major amounts of protein. We use it in place of rice, it's so versatile and tasty, not to mention, great for you! Luckily for Grayson, one thing I have going for me is creativity. So while our ingredients are limited, our diet hasn't been quite so boring. I mix it up a bit and amazingly, since we started this diet, Grayson's cravings (a sign of food allergies) have disappeared and he eats everything!! He wouldn't touch meat with a ten foot pole, now he eats steak, turkey, chicken, pork, fish of all kinds, shellfish, he's eating veggies without a fight, imagine that? A three year old eating veggies and saying he likes them? I make creative pestos for him, he loves garlic which is great for him and adds some umph to his foods, he is very*

interested in spices and cooking with me, so while this has been a challenge, we
are up to it and we are learning and growing from it, and with it!

ALTHOUGH WE HAD incredible gains from just the dietary changes, we were still experiencing many other odd behaviors, like the constant swatting and rubbing his ears and nose. There was a time when we thought it was all related to teething, but he was well beyond teething now and it continued. Lining up cars became his regular past time and obsessions ruled his play.

In combination with working with our local DAN! doctor, we added another DAN! doctor from CA to our team, who was well known in the Autism community. We were guided through various tests which served to solidify our concerns about Grayson's health, his results mirrored those of other children with Autism. We reviewed them with our local DAN! doctor who confirmed our suspicions when all of our insurance paperwork was suddenly coded with **PDD-NOS** (pervasive development disorder not otherwise specified), although we never directly asked for a label. A label can lock you into a box. I have never fit into any boxes and I wasn't going to start now. Getting stuck in a diagnosis can spiral us into horribly unhealthy feelings associated with low vibrations and then we reside right there in those frequencies, unknowingly. Receiving a label for our son wouldn't change who he was to us. I didn't plan on following the mainstream path for Autism which suggested therapy as the only solution. We knew what we were dealing with now. It was time to put on the deep wader boots and jump in feet first.

---

1. Marcello M. DiStasio MD, PhD Ikue Nagakura PhD Monica J. Nadler PhD Matthew P. Anderson MD, PhD, *T-lymphocytes and Cytotoxic Astrocyte Blebs Correlate Across Autism Brains*, First published: 08 October 2019 https://doi.org/10.1002/ana.25610
2. NeuroScience News, First evidence of immune response targeting brain cells in autism, (Oct. 2019), https://neurosciencenews.com/immune-cells-autism-15086/?Âfbclid=IwAR2vrKbENryxIdgrJcHs7shlVkj2qPqkBHVU5DSP2nvi-N5upd41DxSgKDlU

7

Trials and tribulations

A HINT OF DISCOVERY LEADS TO EXPERIMENTATION

"*When there is a will, there is a way.*"

-*Book of the Later Han*

WHEN OUR TESTS concluded that we were dealing with the overgrowth of some nasty pathogens including clostridium, streptococcus, E.coli and candida, we felt like we had no choice but to fight the battle on our hands. I wish someone would have told me then that we would eventually learn that it's our residing vibration that alters our physical body in ways that attracts "like" frequencies, such as pathogens and dis-ease or alternatively, healing and regeneration. The fine line between the physical and spiritual bodies becomes easily blurred here, but this awareness isn't explored until further into our quest. We were guided by allopathic doctors to focus only on the physical body, therefore we created a battlefield within the terrain of our child's intestines by choosing to use antimicrobials to fight the bad guys. We tried a few courses of prescription drugs, but the feeling in my gut reminded me with every dose, that this was against everything I believed in.

More research divulged a slew of natural bacteria and candida fighters. Our initial experimentation with these antimicrobials was slow and confusing in the beginning. We eventually learned what dosages and frequencies he would need to keep the infections at bay. It was daunting to keep up with everything we were giving daily, but if it meant he could live a normal life, we were going to make it happen. I never stopped believing we would beat this. Never.

We were getting pretty comfortable with our new foods although, the list changes regularly when you are new to dietary restrictions. There is a learning curve associated with getting to know hidden foods and potential new problematic foods. It was a work in progress, but then we took it a step further by creating a rotation diet. A rotation diet is when you avoid the foods you use regularly for three days and then rotate them back in for two days. We learned that with leaky gut, it is important to not feed the same foods over and over and over again, because they will develop a sensitivity to the new foods. How awesome is that? Learning that your child is now sensitive to the only foods he could eat? I wasn't having that, so I created a handy little chart that we followed religiously. We tested him a few years later and 10 foods dropped off of his old IgG list and there were no new foods causing problems! We were clearly getting somewhere!

OF COURSE, when things are going smoothly, we like to rock the boat, right? Here is another entry from my blog, about "challenging" foods. Quite simply, a reaction means you must continue to avoid it while no reaction could mean you are clear to add that food back into the diet. No restricted diet would be complete without occasional food challenges, otherwise you are conceding to remain locked into those limited foods endlessly.

Testing, 1, 2, 3

Oh the fun of "challenging" an allergy diet! With a diet like this, comes the trials and tribulations of testing the foods he can't have to be sure he needs to avoid them, also known as challenging the diet. So last night he was eating his quinoa pasta and since he has been doing so well on the diet (which we have been doing since the first week of September now), I thought it would be a good time to try sheep's cheese. Since he tested positive for cow's milk and goat's milk, it was possible that he could handle sheep's cheese, manchego. I grated a tiny bit on top of his pasta and he gobbled it up, of course. He did great this morning with the exception of waking a tad too early with a stuffy nose. I thought we would be in the clear by afternoon. I hauled him off to school in the hopes that he would have yet another good day. Remind me to tell you how far he has come with issues at school since starting this diet!! Well, when I got there to pick him up after school, his teacher came walking out to me...never a good sign, it's like being called to the principal's office. Uh oh, what did he do? She asked me, if we changed something...well now that you mention it, ummmm, can you say CHEESE?! She said that all of his previous behaviors resurfaced today. He has been doing "remarkably" since the diet and today, it was the old Grayson again. Wow, for her to notice that quickly, this diet is the real deal!! I thought it was odd that he would have these problems at school yet he was so well behaved at home this morning. As I headed for home, I immediately began to realize that it was going to be a LONG evening with Dave away on a business trip!! Epsom salts draw out toxins, so before an early bedtime, I soaked him in the tub for a while hoping they would draw out all the nasties so we can have a nice day tomorrow. A new day...

Now THAT THE diet was in place, the antimicrobials were working their wonders and things were going smoothly, I began to research why the food sensitivities, malabsorption issues, leaky gut and gut bugs were there to begin with. It introduced us to a new world of toxin in our environment. And what to my wondering eyes did I learn...my silver fillings were a big problem.

Lo and behold, silver fillings aren't just silver, they include many toxic metals including nickel and mercury...mercury?! But wait, isn't mercury the same metal that the EPA must be called when even minor spills occur? Why would anyone in their right mind put this in our teeth, permanently? I had eight of these bad boys in my mouth! A few of them were pretty large too. To learn that human breast milk tends to attract heavy metals while I was still breast-feeding my baby, was just dandy! Then we add to the load of heavy metals by allowing them to be injected into our babies via vaccinations. All I wanted to know was how do I get it out of my children?! I would deal with my own exposure in due time, but my innocent children were my priority. Heavy metal testing confirmed my fears, both boys were high in heavy metals. Clearly, we would need to address heavy metals, but how?

I researched into the wee hours of the mornings again, comparing the effectiveness and safety of various chelation protocols when I finally made the decision that a safe and effective form of low-dose, oral chelation with supportive supplements, which was created by a Princeton Ph.D biochemist by the name of Andrew Hall Cutler, was the way to go. I really would have preferred to scratch my eyes out with a vegetable peeler, but I felt like I couldn't just leave the mercury in there either, it was undoubtedly not agreeing with my kiddo. At this stage of the game, I didn't know about Homotoxicology or that homeopathy could work for Autism and toxicities, and I hadn't met those key players just yet. So on with A/C chelation we went.

Oh, what fun!! Waking every three hours at night and dosing chelators around the clock through the weekends wasn't my idea of a good time, but we religiously made this happen. For three. Straight. Years.

After a year into it with Grayson, we also included Gavin in the fun since he was done nursing and I knew that he had been served a nice whopping dose of mercury for a year and a half straight. He started to show signs of candida overgrowth. His big toe nail was exceptionally thick and discolored yellow, he developed a red anal ring that rarely went away. He began to have extreme mood swings after having been such a calm and easy going baby. He also developed physical reactions to dairy and soy through my breast milk.

His eczema went away completely when we avoided these foods, but I wanted to eliminate the root of the problem, which at the time, I thought might be the heavy metals. Ultimately, once I had my amalgam fillings replaced by a biological dentist, I started the protocol as well.

8

New territory

LEARNING HOW ONE SIZE DOES NOT FIT ALL, EVEN AMONG SIBLINGS

"I am not discouraged, because every wrong attempt discarded is another step forward."

-Thomas Edison

WHEN IT FELT like Gavin was becoming more difficult behaviorally, it was time to head back to the drawing board. Clearly being gluten-free, casein-free, soy-free and doing chelation while addressing the microbes wasn't cutting it for him. His behavior began to tick off every box on diagnosis lists for ODD (Oppositional Defiance Disorder). This was new territory for us. Our previously sweet, mellow and cuddly baby was now screeching instead of speaking, he was angry much of his awake time, and he even felt totally disconnected at times. Even in a peaceful environment, we couldn't understand why he wanted to hit in response to everything Grayson did within arm's reach of him. He had little to no impulse control and he was aggressive. We decided we should probably run an IgG panel on him, but it resulted in almost nothing telling. He was sensitive to five foods and there was no evidence of gut permeability. What were we dealing with?

I BEGAN READING MORE about dietary restrictions that worked for multiple symptoms he was exhibiting, and when I dug deeper into the Low Oxalate Diet, I felt like it was our next road on the path to wellness. We had done an Organic Acid Test on Grayson years before that resulted in very high oxalic acid numbers, but at the time, we were dealing with so many other highly volatile issues that it went on the back burner. Maybe now was the time to revisit this topic, since it was likely that we were seeing signs of elevated oxalates with our younger son too.

Oxalates are a component of all food, but are more prevalent in plant foods and serve as a natural pesticide for the plant. An example of foods unusually high in oxalate levels are: spinach, chocolate, all nuts, most grains, the skins of most fruits, beets, sweet potatoes and many more. For individuals whose bodies tend to accumulate and store oxalates in an attempt to remove them from circulation in the blood stream, it is imperative that they keep their intake low or they risk potentially painful symptoms related to the excretion of mass quantities of oxalates. It is common for people with fibromyalgia to have elevated oxalate stores and I would encourage anyone with joint pain, at minimum, to check into this possibility. The more common symptoms appear when the person is dumping oxalates, which is an act of the body excreting previously stored oxalates periodically and can consist of any of the following symptoms: skin rashes, sandy feeling stool, burning upon urination, bloating, pain in the urethra, joints, eyes, heart , bones and especially the lower back (when they are accumulating in the kidneys), a common place for oxalates to be stored as the body attempts to pass them through the filtration system of the kidneys.

In fact, the result of oxalates stored in the kidneys is the formation of kidney stones. Once oxalates are stored in the cells, they can interfere with mitochondrial function, causing a severe decrease in energy, and without proper mitochondrial function, your cells will actually starve to death. So, oxalates are essentially natural toxins that the body is attempting to sequester and excrete, but not without deleterious effects in the process.

There are various possible causes for the accumulation of oxalates. It is believed that oxalates accumulate more so when the bacteria that is solely responsible for degrading oxalates, known as Oxalobacter formigenes, is reduced within the intestinal tract. This could be due to: the use of antibiotics, eating processed foods, pesticides, genetically modified and chemical-laden foods which wipe out good bacteria, and could even be related to intestinal infections responsible for gut flora imbalance. The body is capable of converting some substances into oxalates such as Glyphosate, sweeteners and vitamin C. For someone who doesn't realize they have an oxalate issue, IV vitamin C can actually trigger overt oxalate toxicity. Adding insult to injury, leaky gut allows dietary oxalates to enter the blood stream, contributing to a systemic oxalate problem.

It is also believed that mold/fungi and parasites produce oxalates as a byproduct, while depleting the O. formigenes population by sheer existence, contributing to leaky gut. So as you can see, there is a vicious cycle that can ensue, regardless of what causes the problem to begin with. Sadly, because the O. formigenes bacteria is anaerobic, it cannot survive outside of the body, and therefore has not been successfully used in a probiotic product to date, although there are a few companies still attempting to make it happen.

WE DON'T KNOW EXACTLY what triggered our oxalate problem, but when I look back at the timing of everything, I personally developed an oxalate problem after moving into our current home, which did have a mold problem at one time. Gavin was born in this home and Grayson has lived here since he was two and a half, which is also when his symptoms picked up speed. The only thing I know for certain is that we don't have the markers for the inherited genetic disorder known as Hyperoxaluria, which causes the body to actually make oxalates endogenously, potentially causing renal failure as the body tries to eliminate the oxalates through the kidneys. In the case of Hyperoxaluria, the liver doesn't create enough of a certain enzyme that prevents the overproduction of oxalate, or the enzyme doesn't work properly. Regardless of the cause, when a person has oxalate build up, it isn't something to be taken lightly, because cell death has the ability to effect all functions in the body.

As WE BEGAN to reduce higher oxalate foods in the boys' diets, their specific symptoms associated with oxalates were glaring. When dietary intake is reduced, intra-cellular oxalates begin to leave the body, and fast, especially if you reduce dietary oxalates too fast. This is what is known as having an oxalate "dump." We trudged painstakingly through eight weeks of oxalate dumping symptoms. Our poor little guy experienced random joint pains, an aching lower back, sleepless nights, eye pains (he poked at them attempting to ease the pains), painful urination and sandy stools, as well as horrible mood swings.

Gavin had been potty learning without much success for so long, and was still having accidents frequently. It was baffling, because we almost had him entirely trained, yet when we were out of the house he could often control it, but at home he was still experiencing a lot of accidents. We thought he was just too busy playing to break for the potty when he was home.

WITHIN THREE WEEKS of going low oxalate, he was fully trained! It was an eye-opener for us when we experienced his first of many potties full of oxalate crystals. Lowering oxalates in the diet initiates oxalate "dumping" which produces symptoms associated with the oxalate accumulation leaving the body. We would never have noticed this if he was using a full sized toilet instead of his little plastic training toilet. One afternoon, I was in a hurry to get some-where and in order to avoid spending all of our time visiting public rest rooms, I always asked my boys go to the bathroom before leaving the house. On this day, I didn't have time to empty Gavin's toilet before running out the door. He just did a little tinkle and we left. I would deal with it later. After putting them to bed, I went to clean his potty and was astonished when I found his potty bowl (which was red) lined with tons of white, sharp-looking crystals, also known as oxalates!! All I could think of was, "Ouch! That must have hurt coming out!" It was confirming that we were on the right path though, that's for sure.

9

Necessary evil

REMOVING HEAVY METALS FROM THE BODY DOESN'T COME WITHOUT RISK, BUT LEAVING THEM THERE DOES

"Y ou cannot swim for new horizons until you have courage to lose sight of the shore."

-William Faulkner

CHELATION IS the process of of liberating heavy metals from their stored locations in the body by introducing a chelator into the system, with the intent of helping the body flush these heavy metals. Sounds easy enough, right? Just get them out so we can move on. But no, it's not that easy. There is a whole lot more to think about in order to accomplish safe detoxification.

There are a number of different chelators. Some are used intravenously by doctors in very high doses. Many are naturally sourced, which sounds ideal, but too many of the natural chelators are more successful at liberating metals then they are at eliminating them. Anytime heavy metals are mobilized, they enter the blood stream, creating symptoms in their wake. One of the downsides of chelation therapy, even while using safer chelators, is the inevitable disruption of the microbiome. Pathogenic microbes use heavy metals as food, causing temporary overgrowth, which then needs to be controlled in order to prevent the cascade of pathogenic endotoxins flooding the system and ultimately the detox organs.

The chelator must be capable of not only liberating the metals from stored tissue and cells, but also binding with them tightly enough to help the body excrete them appropriately, otherwise they could just move around and find a new storage location. I personally don't take this lightly, because of the potential to redistribute heavy metals.

When we began supplementation with natural oral chelators to remove heavy metals, we had no idea how intense the process would be, how hard it would be on the body, or how trying it would be for our family as a result. All we knew was that we were heavy metal toxic and we would never take the risk of IV chelation, which sits too high up on the risky scale for my taste. Low oral dosing with supplemental chelators seemed like a necessary, but lesser evil. Knowing it could take years to be fully effective weighed on us, but I was determined to do whatever it took to safely heal our family. Heavy metal accumulation combined with a decreased ability to effectively detox contributes to many chronic conditions, including Autism.

ROLLING over and wondering if we missed the last chelator dose, I nudged Dave, *"The alarm is going off, Dave…"*

Did I just sleep through Dave getting up only three hours ago? He dragged his weary body out of bed for the second time tonight to dose the kids with their chelation supplements while I turned over wracking my brain to remember if I took my own dose three hours ago. The clock was blurry, but in my usual organized way, I had devised a plan so I wouldn't lose track. I reached my heavy hand into the little cup on the night stand which held my three overnight doses, Two left, good I took the first capsule. I often didn't even remember dosing myself these midnight rounds of chelators.

Missing a dose meant having to stop the round and wait for the next round to resume, because the pattern of dosing would be broken and the half-life of the chelator would expire. The reason for the timely dosing is related to maintaining a steady level of a low-dose, oral chelator in the blood stream which results in a continuous flow of excreted heavy metals. As soon as the half- life of the chelator expires, metals begin to drop into the blood stream where they have the potential to redistribute. Redistribution allows them to attach to tissues and organs.

Unfortunately, this is inevitable with each round of chelation, regardless of how small of a dose is being used. By maintaining the 3-4 hour dosing schedule, redistribution only occurs once, only when each round ends. By keeping the doses VERY low, the effects are minimal.

I can honestly say, I felt GREAT during chelation most of the time, there was clarity and calm. In between rounds, I felt a slump in my days. Even with the progress we experienced, years of waking all night long to keep up with the demands of the process took its toll on us long term. We were chronically exhausted, and we didn't know which symptoms were pure exhaustion and which were pathogenic overgrowth.

SIX MONTHS after having my amalgams replaced by a Huggin's approved biological dentist, I began to experience what is commonly referred to as "the six month [mercury] dump." Andrew Cutler's research uncovered a pattern to the natural detox of mercury from the body. First, it leaves the bloodstream for several months, then the organs begin to dump their mercury. At this stage, blood and urine mercury levels actually increase. This means there is a fabulous honeymoon period for a few months and then around six months the dumping is at its highest, meaning...I was at my worst! Supplemental, low-dose chelation is supposed to greatly reduce this effect. I can only imagine what my experience might have been like if I wasn't softening the blow! There were days when I could equate what I felt like to Autism. It was during this period when I also felt my best during the weekend rounds on chelation, because the free-floating mercury was actively being escorted out.

"Damn it!!" I mumbled under my breath, as I watched the $165 bottle of Custom Probiotics fall towards my tile floor. At first, it seemed to be in slow motion, that is, until the startling sound of the shattering jar billowed through the house.

"What was that, Mommy?" Grayson called from the family room.

"Oh nothing, I just dropped something." I retorted, while still standing there glaring at the mess it made. As I cleaned the shards of glass that slid under the pantry door, I glanced up at my calendar to see the words I had written six months earlier, *"6 month dump!"* I was right smack in the middle of it. Joy!

I had been fumbling through so many clumsy accidents lately. My mood swings were wild too. There was no buffer between calm and furious. Even worse, I had no remorse. Instead, I just wanted to run away. Better yet, truth be known, I wanted everyone else to run away and leave me in my bedroom to wallow in misery. I would have been happy sleeping all day long. I couldn't even carry on a full conversation. Words hovered around in the space above my head, rarely making their way to my mouth without effort. Anyone who knows me, knows that I like to talk, and words generally come easy for me! It was as if my brain and mouth were no longer connected, there was a detour right where the words were created. What worried me most was the degree of anger I was experiencing. It flipped on like a switch with no warning. It surprised even me! I really began to understand Autism from a totally different perspective, from the inside. Thankfully, the severity of these symptoms faded within a few months.

I BEGAN to wonder when the chelation nightmare would ever end. Three years and counting, and we still couldn't reduce the antimicrobials that kept the gut bugs under control. In fact, it felt like we were being driven to increase them over time, because the candida and bacterial symptoms were off the charts. Although we felt like chelation had definitely sparked improvement in the beginning, it wasn't appearing to effect much any longer, other than to instigate the gut bugs. We had invested so much faith and time into the process that we weren't sure if we could just back out so easily, but after a lengthy break during a few back-to-back illnesses, we just never went back to it. That was my confirmation that we were meant to move on.

10

Let's try this again

TRUSTING THE WISDOM OF HOMEOPATHY

"The highest ideal of cure is the speedy, gentle, and enduring restoration of health by the most trustworthy and least harmful way."

-Samuel Hahnemann, founder of homeopathy

Shortly before our final departure from chelation, we had begun working with a new doctor, who was also a homeopath, in an attempt to weave homeopathy into our routine with the kids. You may recall that we briefly tried a few homeopathic remedies after Grayson's vaccine reactions, without much success. It was, however, undeniably successful for me and had been in the back of my mind ever since. I knew we would give it another try "sometime soon."

When I found a local doctor who focused primarily on homeopathy, we felt confident in our decision to consult with her. She fused the two worlds we were straddling, the holistic and the conventional.

This doctor practiced a form of classical homeopathy that consisted of using a single remedy long-term. She thought chelation therapy might create a block in healing, but was willing to see how treatment could progress concurrently.

We had a clear and undeniable response to Grayson's first dose of his prescribed remedy! Chelation clearly wasn't completely blocking healing, but could it interfere with long-term results? Only time would tell.

I STILL REMEMBER that first dose like it was yesterday. He had just been evaluated for SPD where it was determined that his style of descending on the stairs had to do with his delayed gross motor skills development. He would always lead with his right foot, which would then be slowly and cautiously met by his left foot, then he would repeat it, right foot, met by left, all while holding the railing tightly, as if he would fall without it. We gave the first dose of his remedy in the evening when we got home from the appointment and he went off to bed. The very next morning, he came running down the stairs to me...RUNNING! No holding the railing, no feet meeting on the steps...running, one foot after the other. I was so stunned, I asked him to return to the top of the stairs and repeat it, which he proudly did for me.

WRAPPING your head around the quantum physics associated with homeopathy and energy medicine requires you to leave behind what you think you know about medicine and science. Homeopathy is a 200-year-old system of medicine based on a principle that "like cures like," also known as the Law of Similars. Believe it or not, vaccines were actually an attempt at utilizing this concept, although poorly applied and with destructive, crude material doses of dangerous ingredients. We are not actually anti-vaccine as much as we are just anti-dangerous-ingredients, but show me a vaccine that doesn't have dangerous ingredients in it, and I will show you a vaccine I trust. I encourage you to run through a list of vaccine ingredients from the packaging insert (which can all be found online now) and research a handful of them individually. The inherent risk will become all too glaring as soon as you do a little homework. Homeopathy, on the other hand, has the capacity to prevent and treat dis-ease without the added burden of the risk of harm.

When the founder of homeopathy, Dr. Samuel Hahnemann (1755-1843), first applied this principle to medicine, it was because he was disenchanted by the harmful medical practices of his day. Homeopathy is gentle, in that it operates by influencing the vital force, encouraging the body to heal itself. The vital force is analogous to the theory of qi in Chinese medicine, or prana in Ayurveda: it is the energy of life. What may appear to be a small detail is actually the very difference between a living and a non-living body.

Homeopathy is aimed at healing the vital force rather than just eliminating the symptoms, as modern medicine has taken to doing. Proof of this vital force has been seen in photos taken with a camera that was developed by the Kirlians, also known as Kirlian Photography. Changes in energy patterns were documented in various states of health and death. With decreasing life energy, life itself dies.

In ninth grade science, I recall learning about how everything has its own totally unique frequency, a rate at which it vibrates. My teacher lifted an apple off of a student's desk and announced that the apple in his hand vibrated at a different frequency than the desk, which he knocked on with his other hand, and that they both had a different vibration from the frequency of the dusty chalkboard behind him.

IN "A NEW EARTH," Eckhart Tolle describes this phenomenon:

> *"The chair you sit on, the book you are holding in your hands appear solid and motionless only because that is how your senses perceive their vibrational frequency, that is to say, the incessant movement of the molecules, atoms, electrons and subatomic particles that together create what you perceive as a chair, a book, a tree or a body. What we perceive as physical matter is energy vibrating (moving) at a particular range of frequencies. Thoughts consist of the same energy vibration at a higher frequency than matter, which is why they*

cannot be seen or touched. Thoughts have their own range of frequencies, with negative thoughts at the lower end of the scale and positive thoughts at the higher."

Everything, including illnesses and emotions, have their own vibrational thumbprint. It's these frequencies which homeopathy interacts with. When a vibrational frequency is stimulated by a similar frequency, it will increase. In "The Science of Homeopathy" to describe the concept of resonance, homeopath George Vithoulkas shared the example of a tuning fork. When one tuning fork is struck, another across the room will vibrate in resonance to the first one. The vital force responds to and adjusts with every stimulus it is exposed to. Typically the body can manage most minor stimuli, however, if the stimulus' strength is stronger than the vital force itself, it is compelled to adjust in a way that the consequences become tangible in the mind, body and spirit.

FOR A MORE SPECIFIC understanding of how homeopathic remedies appear to work, I will need to explain how they are made, because it's in the making of the remedy where the real magic happens. While critics have suggested there is "nothing in them," laboratory experiments have demonstrated that homeopathic remedies are not just sugar pills. In fact, Dr. E.S. Rajendran, teacher, researcher and practicing homeopath in India has personally discovered nanoparticles in homeopathic remedies ranging from 6C to CM potencies! So while medical professionals will have you believing there is nothing in these sugar pellets beyond the potency of 12C, Dr. Rajendran has actually confirmed that just one drop of a remedy contains many millions of nano-particles in the range of 1-10nm using High- Resolution Transmission Electron Microscopy (HRTEM), Field Emission Scanning Electron Microscopy (FESEM) and spectroscopy measurements (a way of identifying what atoms are present in a sample in a particular location). He proved that the nano-particulate quantum dots contain atoms from the parent-material. For example, the remedy Aurum Metallicum which is made from gold, contains the presence of gold in the quantum dots. The higher the potency, the finer the particles observed. The finer the particle, the more easily absorbed they are, yet the parent-material's toxicity is eliminated. So while the science of this 200-year-old medicine is still evolving with the times, the effectiveness remains the same. And the particulate matter of homeopathy confirms without a doubt, that homeopathy IS evidence-based medicine![1]

IN DR. RAJENDRAN's own words,

> *"Homeopathy is advanced, it produces epigenetic modification, it cures disease at a genetic level. Modern medicine is mostly a biomolecular medicine, it goes to the biochemical level, in general."*

Those of us using homeopathy religiously don't need the studies to prove what we have witnessed in our own family members, but if you haven't been blessed with your own personal experience with homeopathy, this should be of interest to you.

ACCORDING to the Homeopathic Research Institute,

> *"Some homeopathic medicines are diluted beyond the threshold known as Avogadro's number (dilution 10-23). This means that the liquid is so highly diluted that you would not expect any molecules of the original substance to remain.*
>
> *It is these 'ultra-high dilutions' (homeopathic medicines above 12c or 24x potency) which attract controversy, because they clearly cannot work in the same way as conventional medical drugs, i.e. through molecules interacting directly with the body's biochemistry. Researchers around the world are investigating the mechanism of action of these medicines, which is likely to be based in physics rather than chemistry. Although there are various theories being explored, as yet, we do not understand how homeopathic medicines work.*
>
> *What we do know is that many laboratory studies have shown ultra-high*

dilution homeopathic medicines having biological effects that you would not see if they were 'just water' or 'just sugar pills', for example:

Adding homeopathic histamine to basophils (white blood cells) can trigger them to release histamine and Homeopathic thyroxine, at the dilution of 30x, slows down the rate at which tadpoles turn into frogs.

The key appears to be in exactly how homeopathic medicines are made

Homeopathic medicines are made from plant, chemical, mineral or animal sources. The original material is diluted, then agitated vigorously (succussed). The number of times this is repeated determines the strength or 'potency' of the remedy e.g. a '6c' remedy will have been diluted 1 part in 100 then succussed, six times over.

If you only dilute the substance over and over, of course you are eventually left with an inactive sample which is 'just water'; it is the added succussion between each step of dilution which appears to imprint information from the original substance, into the water/ alcohol it is diluted in.

This idea is supported by experiments which show that unsuccussed dilutions are inactive, but succussed dilutions can cause biological effects, suggesting that this aspect of the manufacturing process is essential in creating homeopathic medicines." [2]

YOU MAY ALREADY KNOW that water holds memory, and when you put a substance into water, then succuss and dilute it as described above, the water takes on the molecular shape and spin of that substance while diluting the material dose, eliminating the toxic qualities, thereby creating a new substance that mimics the original substance. This new substance, which acts like the original substance, contains all of the benefits but none of the harm (the higher the potency, the finer the particles, as described above). So when you use a homeopathic remedy like Arsenicum (made from arsenic), you will not be poisoned by the remedy, because the particles (quantum dots, to be exact) are undetectable without an electron microscope. Now you are able to experience the beneficial qualities of a substance that would otherwise be dangerous to ingest.

· · ·

I'D LIKE to provide more of a visual based on my own research and understanding of how the act of dilution and succussion work. Let's look at an example using snake venom, also known as Lachesis muta in homeopathy.

The remedy is made from the venom of the Bushmaster snake, one of the largest and most dangerous snakes in South America. In its crude material form, if you were to encounter this snake venom, it would be deadly, correct? Within 5 hours of a bite, you would develop symptoms such as edema, pain, hemorrhage, blister formation at the site of the bite, bradycardia, diminished heart function, loss of consciousness, blurry vision, vomiting and possibly other serious reactions. This is because snake venom is poisonous, but when you create a homeopathic remedy with this very venom, it is no longer poisonous, and that secret is in the creation of the remedy.

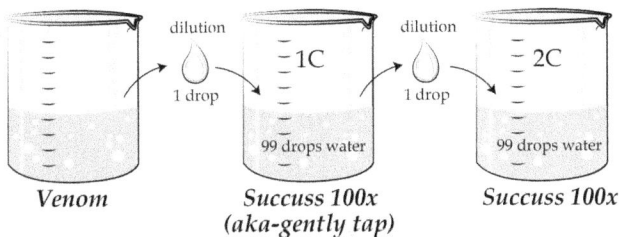

dilution   dilution

1 drop   1C   1 drop   2C

99 drops water   99 drops water

Venom   *Succuss 100x*   *Succuss 100x*
                 (aka-gently tap)

and so on to create
30 c
200 c
1000 c (1M)
10,000c (10M)
50,000 c (50M)

To make homeopathic Lachesis muta, one single drop of the venom is added to 99 drops of purified water. When this solution is succussed, as mentioned above, the water molecules (which have memory) take on the molecular spin of the venom, meaning that now the water itself is mimicking the molecular behavior of the venom. But if you were to drink this, there may still be enough venom in the solution to be poisonous. As mentioned by the Home-

opathy Research Institute above, we will need to create a 12C
remedy to alter enough of the original molecules of the venom in
the remedy to render it "undetectable" by medical standards, in
other words, safe. Although, I've used many lower potency remedies
made from poisonous substances without ill effect.

In order to stay on track, I won't get into this too deeply (there
are other great books for this). There are multiple scales of potencies to homeopathic remedies, they are X, C, M and LM. The dilution and succussion counts used to create each potency are as
follows: 10 for X, 100 for C, 1000 for M and LM potencies are a bit
more complicated because they are derived from 3C potencies, but
are more highly diluted initially. I won't confuse you with a full
explanation of the LM potencies.

Now we know that one hundred dilutions and succussions are
needed to create a 1C remedy, to go on to a 2C, we repeat this
process and use one drop of the 1C remedy which is added to 99
drops of purified water and then succussed another one hundred
times.

Refer back to the diagram for the visual image.

TO RECAP FOR CLARITY:

- 1 drop of crude venom added to 99 drops of water then
  100 succussions = 1C
- 1 drop of 1C solution added to 99 drops of water then
  100 succussions = 2C
- 1 drop of 2C solution added to 99 drops of water then
  100 succussions = 3C
- And so on...

This process is repeated for each potency in the "C" scale. To
reach 12C, it is completed 12 times, for a total of 12 dilutions and
1200 succussions. The crude doses of the venom are no longer
detectable at this potency, yet the water maintains the molecular
structure of the original poisonous venom and through this

process, only nanoparticles remain. In a homeopathic pharmacy, this process is done with grain alcohol, which is then dropped onto sugar pellets where they will hold the information from the alcohol. The sugar pellets act as a carrier of the information from millions of atoms in the alcohol. When the remedy is taken, this frequency or vibration of the venom is being expressed from the remedy and it is now able to neutralize any of the above symptoms (and others) that the crude poisonous venom would cause, which his referred to as the Law of Similars or "like cures like." The Law of Similars says that a substance that will produce symptoms in a healthy person can actually cure those same symptoms in an ill person. The imprint of the symptoms is essentially neutralized when a corresponding remedy match is accurately determined.

Just as the homeopathic remedy retains the imprint of the original substance, let's consider that a human body is made up of more than 70% water (with many of the organs being made up of over 90% water), so when a trauma occurs, that trauma becomes imprinted on the body, very much like a homeopathic remedy holds the imprint of the original substance. It is not diluted and succused, but the raw imprint exists none the less. The concept of like cures like, also known as the Law of Similars means that we will actually be able to neutralize this imprint on the body, with a remedy of matching vibration. This is, in effect, the basis of the work done by a professional homeopath.

As you know, you don't have to have been bitten by a snake to experience some of the symptoms I listed earlier, which also means you could use Lachesis for any indications that look similar, as long as there are a few rubrics (the homeopathic term for symptom) in the remedy that match them, and the etiology (the cause or set of causes) of the remedy matches the situation. Homeopathic remedies each have hundreds, if not thousands, of indicating symptoms that effect the physical, mental and spiritual realm of the being. So you can imagine there is a lot more taken into account for the prescription of a homeopathic remedy intended to treat a chronic illness. It is recommended that if you would like to undertake homeopathic treatment for a chronic condition, you hire a homeopath who is trained in the principals of healing according the Law of Similars.

HOMEOPATHY WORKS *with* the healing mechanism of the body by supporting its innate responses. If the body wants to create inflammation at the site of a burn for the purpose of healing tissue damage at the burn site, the homeopathic remedy chosen will reflect a key component of inflammation, to help the body respond appropriately and faster. For centuries, homeopathy has proven to reduce and eliminate tumors, heal aching limbs, reverse nutritional deficiencies, speed up recoveries of all kinds, treat and prevent epidemics and even eliminate pain of all kinds, without causing harm in the process. I bet you are wondering why doctors all over aren't using it, if it works so well. Because the pharmaceutical industry is a major money-making business. There were homeopathic hospitals in just about every state at one time. If you go down the rabbit-hole of how that changed, you will find pharmaceuticals (namely antibiotics) at the root of its demise.

THANKFULLY, homeopathy is still a medical art that is available and it's worth the investment. My opinion, contrary to what anyone believes, is that it WILL work for anyone and everyone, as long as they find the right practitioner match for their situation. There are literally dozens of different styles of treatment and on one hand, and this is great, because it offers numerous options, however, it can also create a dizzying effect when you are navigating the recovery of one's health.

Homeopathy treats the patient as a whole. Modern medicine has made a habit of compartmentalizing illness by separating the symptom/organ from the whole being. There are doctors specialized in the gastrointestinal tract, others specialized in mental illness, others for the heart, and so on. By suggesting they are specialized in their field, we are lead to believe that they know everything there is to know about that organ, but what about how it interacts with the other organs in the body? For example, when the intestinal tract is inflamed, this can result in mental symptoms, because half of our neurotransmitters are in our intestines. A person experiencing mental illness might not know to consider their gastrointestinal health and could end up going to a psychiatrist who will ultimately put this person on mind altering drugs, in an attempt to deal with the mental disturbances the only way he knows how.

The personal and particular expressions of illness can be witnessed in all illnesses. Let's take the example of the common cold. Two people can contract the same virus, yet the symptoms they exhibit may be completely different. One person might have symptoms of a runny nose, itchy skin, diarrhea and they might feel better when they drink ice water, but worse from being covered in blankets and warmth. The second person may have symptoms of bloating and constipation, dry lips and mouth, a splitting headache and they could feel better drinking warm drinks and made worse by fresh air. The mind, body and spirit are interdependent forces, they are united. Kirlian photography has confirmed through images that in a healthy state, the mind, body and spirit remain in balance. If, however, the vital force is disturbed, they become imbalanced eventually resulting in illness or dis-case and symptoms ultimately develop in the physical body.

TRAUMA CREATES a negative imprint on the vital force and that negative imprint causes pathological problems. An old knee injury is healed up physically, but the memory, the impression on the vital body at the site of the knee injury causes that knee to be weaker than the other knee. We must treat the mind, body and spirit together in order to see unified balance return. The chosen homeopathic remedy must be just as individual as the person. Homeopathic case taking is quite a lengthy process, which unravels the many unique characteristic layers of the patient, therefore, ideal remedy matches are essential to healing. Healing may take place on a zig zag path over a number of years, or less frequently, with a perfect one-time match, but the right remedies are critical none the less.

WE'VE BEEN BRAINWASHED to think symptoms are "bad," because we have associated them with illness and "needing" a doctor to help us heal. If we have a runny nose or a fever, we believe something bad is going on in our bodies and we are driven to eliminate the symptoms in order to feel as though we are well again, although the elimination of symptoms often times doesn't equate to health. In actuality, symptoms are the result of our body healing whatever is imbalanced in the body. They are a sign that the body is doing what it is designed to do, heal itself! Examples of this are seen in sneezing, which is a simple act of expelling a foreign invader from the nostrils, be it a microbe or an allergen. A fever increases the core body temperature just enough to kill off pathogenic microbes which can't live in this elevated temperature. Inflammation is the process where the body sends the appropriate blood cells to the injured site to repair the damage, as well as preventing more damage from occurring.

When these symptoms don't retreat or they are suppressed regularly by the use of medications that just temporarily eliminate the symptoms themselves, we refer to this as a chronic disease. This chronic disease state is a red flag, hailing us to make a change in our lifestyle. It means something isn't right and the body isn't able to recover from the onslaught of toxins invading our body.

TO UNDERSTAND a little more about how homeopathy works in contrast to allopathic medication, it is important to understand how the body heals itself, as well as how the body communicates the functions it uses to heal itself. The actions above (and more) are dictated by a complex system going on beneath your skin. Our bodies maintain a unique system of communication. How do the right blood cells find their way to the injured site in order to heal it? How does our thyroid know it's time to release thyroxin? How do certain microbes know to fight off invaders? What is it that our body does to communicate the many essential tasks that keep us alive? The answers lie in the science of physics, where we can learn about frequencies and electromagnetic signals.

Frequency is the measurable rate of electrical energy flow that is constant between any two points. As mentioned earlier, everything has frequency. Our cells are like little batteries, conducting electricity. The nervous system uses electrical energy, also known as nerve impulses, to transmit messages from one cell to another. Imbalances of any of these ions, or inhibition of ion transport across the cell membranes, can lead to dysfunction in the conduction of electrical messages. This dysfunction quickly leads to a general body disturbance and loss of energetic stability in the bio-field of our body. Additionally, this dysfunction skews internal messaging between the cells, blocks conduction of electrical messages in the nervous system and can alter or change electromagnetic signals in the body.

The heart is an electromagnetic organ, in fact, it is detectible enough to be measured with an instrument that measures EMF in the environment. Our DNA sequences emit low frequency electromagnetic waves which make up DNA signals that organize the nucleotides, or arrange the pattern of raw material. Microbes also communicate via frequencies, in fact, some of the most successful treatments for antibiotic resistant strains of pathogenic microbes use a frequency that interrupts their communication.

According to Dr. Robert O. Becker in his book "The Body Electric," the human body has an electrical frequency and much about a person's health can be determined by it. Dr. Royal R. Rife found that every disease has a frequency. He found that certain frequencies can prevent the development of disease and that others would destroy diseases.

Substances of higher frequency will destroy diseases of lower frequency. The information on how the body relies on frequencies is endless, so it goes without saying that the use of frequencies within the body is a form of speaking its own language, and the results can be quite profound. Homeopathy does just that. Homeopathic remedies are literally doses of frequencies which communicate with the body on a level that is quite hard for most practitioners to comprehend, but is in complete alignment with how our bodies work.

I⟩ was a relief that we had finally pulled the trigger on homeopathy and were seeing results so quickly this time around. It was evident that the right remedy makes all the difference. Now, that we had officially decided not to continue with chelation for other reasons, we were free to explore this modality more fully and without fear of interfering with healing by using potentially conflicting modalities.

---

1. Nanoparticles in homeopathy - Prof (Dr). ES Rajendran MD (Hom) PhD research papers - http://www.esrajendran.com/publications.html#researchPaper
2. "There's nothing in it, just sugar pills - Laboratory experiments have demonstrated that homeopathic medicines are not just sugar pills" https://www.hri-research.org/resources/homeopathy-faqs/theres-nothing-in-it-its-just-sugar-pills/

11

Meditation does what?

"*The quieter you become, the more you can hear.*"

-Ram Dass

GROWING UP, I had a pretty intense personality. I stressed easily and projected my tension onto others by attempting to prove myself right to anyone who disagreed with my views. You can imagine how uptight that would make a person. I often blurted out facts or anecdotes to support my firmly held beliefs, without much compassion for my opponent's perspective, leaving many people frustrated, uncomfortable and sometimes even exhausted in my wake.

FOR SUCH A LEFT-BRAINED, analytical person though, I spent an awful lot of my spare time engaged in right-brained activities like writing poetry, painting, drawing and creating. I could usually be found alone in my room singing along with some moody, alternative female artist while my creativity flowed into my art. My family discovered very early on that I didn't like to be interrupted when I was deeply involved. This takes me back to when I was just eleven or twelve years old. I had been out in the backyard deeply involved in a watercolor painting.

From around the corner of the house, I hear my mother calling excitedly for me, her volume increasing as she advances closer, *"Jeeeess….Jess, oh there you are! Someone is here to see you!"*

And with that, a boy from school shyly approaches the table where I am painting and asks if I'd like to go for a walk with him. My mother was visibly excited for me as she tried to busy herself nearby.

My response…callously, and without even lifting my eyes from my painting, I manage a curt, *"I'm busy."*

My mother was appalled. She was and still is a very social butterfly. She couldn't believe I would choose painting alone over taking a walk with a "nice boy." To this day, I couldn't even tell you that boy's name. I hope he isn't reading this book!

IT's apparent to me now, in hindsight, that my hobbies were an organic attempt to balance and calm my central nervous system. Just like sitting in meditation, when I was in that state of focus, nothing could get to me.

It wasn't until we had Grayson that both Dave and I recognized that we didn't have a structured belief system to raise him from. Parents need a backbone of inspiration to help visualize their values and morals, as a vehicle for infusing the family culture with a strong foundation. Neither of us followed any one religion, but both of us desired connection with something greater than us. We both felt drawn to Universal knowing in some way and often had profound intellectual discussions about the mysteries of the world. Those conversations were part of the strong bond we developed early in our relationship. We knew we saw eye to eye, but we didn't identify with it as religion. It's not that we hadn't been raised with religious influences, both of us had minor, but available religious resources. We just didn't connect deeply with them, and when the discussion of baptism came up for Grayson, we both felt sorely underprepared for the weight of choosing this path for another human.

Having had an innate interest in the Orient and frequently reading about Buddhism and Taoism growing up, I felt a distant, but very powerful magnetism to Buddhism that took me decades to cultivate into lifestyle. Without even realizing it, Dave and I *had* already begun a life together based on a common belief system, we just hadn't identified with it yet. Our lifestyle evolved and became more clear to us while researching and experimenting with a multitude of alternative-healing modalities that were rooted in the Far East.

I found myself at home with meditation and yoga. Both had the uncanny ability to instantly connect me with my purpose. No matter what challenges I was confronted with, meditation and yoga had the capacity to re-center my energy without fail, allowing me to hone in with laser accuracy on what's important in that moment. Regular yoga followed by even a short meditation, grounds me in ways nothing else can. I experience a unique stability that doesn't exist otherwise.

I instinctually began diving deeper and deeper into the depths of my intuition and forming a trusting bond with myself. Although this newfound confidence was unfamiliar to me, I can say looking back now, that I sense a recognizable reminder of my youth. There is something parallel in the way yoga and meditation center me, like the arts always did. You might just find me listening to some of the same music I was inspired by in my teens! Pairing yoga and meditation with soul-inspiring music elevates the experience ten-fold and my art was always equally motivated by the right music.

With a more neutral start to my days, I was beginning to accept and overcome challenges with less reactivity. I felt less inclined to confront people and more likely to enjoy listening rather than talking. Don't get me wrong, I didn't lose my conviction, I just began to channel it very differently.

. . .

Although it would still be a while before I could say I had this part of me fine-tuned and consistent, it was obvious to me that yoga and meditation (which I tend to do together) were profound players in our health journey. I say "our" journey because a mother sets the tone for her family. If I'm frayed and impatient, so are the kids. If I can't cope with the unexpected nuances of life, how can I expect the rest of the family to respond to me? It's a domino effect.

With the grounded side of me growing stronger with practice, I was exhibiting and modeling ways to calmly and systematically approach our day-to-day struggles. Life looks very different through balanced lenses.

How can meditation help us with Autism, PANDAS/PANS?

Occasionally, a study comes out from a well-respected group of researchers, linking Autism to a deficiency or some other single-handed "cause." While I appreciate the efforts and attempts to identify the cause of Autism, which really does need to be explored and documented, these studies are often as narrow-minded as the conventional treatments themselves. Hopefully, somewhere along the way, the findings can be pulled together and reviewed more holistically, because it is never just one cause or just one body system. All dis-eases are multifaceted and Autism is no exception, therefore it also requires a multi- faceted set of solutions.

One example is a recent promising study from researchers at MIT and Harvard who found a link between a behavioral symptom of Autism and reduced activity of a neurotransmitter whose job is to dampen neuron excitation.[1] This neurotransmitter they are referring to is GABA (gamma aminobutyric acid), which is balanced by yet another neurotransmitter known as glutamate which can be found in many foods and preservatives like MSG. Together, GABA and glutamate are intimately responsible for a whole slew of functions seen in a healthy body. When this balance is tipped in either direction, the resulting symptoms are some of the many cascading events leading to the symptoms we call Autism.

Glutamate is responsible for learning, attending and functioning and increased glutamate receptors are associated with neurologic disorders like Lou Gehrig's Disease, or Amyotrophic Lateral Sclerosis (ALS), Fragile X, Schizophrenia and seizure disorders. One way to keep glutamate under control is to eliminate eating gluten and casein. Increased glutamate causes decreased eye contact, and insomnia and can lead to bladder contraction, strabismus and self-stimulatory behaviors (stims).

GABA on the other hand, which opposes glutamate, has a calming effect. One of the ways the brain deals with excitotoxin damage (caused by elevated glutamates) is to increase the level of opioids which are opium-like substances. They too interfere with the ability to function. As you can see, the GABA-glutamate dance is just one of the many functions we rely on to remain healthy and its resulting imbalances have taken on the shape of the disorder we have come to know as Autism.

When a study compartmentalizes these symptoms and the diseases associated with them for the purpose of creating yet another drug, rather than focusing on why it's happening and how we can holistically resolve the imbalances, I am further discouraged by the "science."

LET'S look at a simple way to increase natural GABA, which in turn will decrease and help balance glutamate levels, without the use of a synthetic substance like drugs or even supplements!

Enter stage left - meditation. To a novice, meditation might resemble an activity for those with intense will power and dedication to calm. Visions of Monks and Buddhists probably come to mind. It's true, they are some of the few who practice meditation on a regular basis and you might even think it's purely a religious practice, but meditation is growing in practice around the globe. It is a practice of mindfulness with far-reaching benefits to human health and wellness. Meditation can be achieved by anyone and everyone, of all ages and lifestyles, and the effects have even been studied and proven by scientists around the world as well. One of the many benefits of meditation is, you guessed it, an increase in the calming neurotransmitter GABA! Psychiatrists at Boston University found a 27% increase in GABA levels after 60 minutes of mindful exercises.[2] That is quite significant, especially if you partake in mindful practices like yoga, Qigong, meditation, and even regular mindful breathing. Meditation boosts serotonin, the happiness neurotransmitter, reduces cortisol which is a major age-accelerating hormone, dramatically boosts DHEA, known to researchers as the "longevity molecule" and raises endorphins, which are responsible for that "feel good effect." So a little bit of meditation goes a long way in terms of health and wellness. This could be just the thing our children need.

I know the next question on your mind is, "How do you encourage your children to meditate?" First and foremost, by modeling it!! We must, must, must model what we expect from our children. It doesn't always come with immediately visible results, but with time and patience, modeling behaviors does inevitably impact our impressionable children. Don't expect to see your children hop onto the floor with you the first time they see you mindfully breathing or meditating, but do share your experiences and DO practice patience here.

One way to start is by verbalizing when you are using this technique. A simple way to do that is when you have encountered something stressful. You can breathe audibly and deeply while expressing that you are frustrated with something and how your deep breathing is going to center your mind and body so you can think clearly.

A great program that teaches children how to understand and use mindfulness techniques is called "MindUp!" You can simply buy the age-appropriate workbooks online and read through them together, then practice the activities together. This will allow you to explain exactly what is taking place in different parts of the brain. The book series starts with preschool aged concepts and runs straight through adolescence, it's VERY helpful in the overall lesson of mindfulness. The activities are also fun!

Another book that would be highly beneficial for the kids who show interest in meditation when you don't know where to begin is called "Sensational Meditation for Children" by Sarah Wood Vallely. Sarah walks you through guided imagery and meditation techniques step by step. You literally read out loud to the children while they envision and experience the meditations as you speak to them. It is interactive, silly and engaging, and you will learn things about your children (and yourself, if you join them). There are fourteen guided meditations to choose from, each with its own unique twist and purpose. My kids especially loved Fudge Swirl, Happy Tree and The Time Machine meditations. The book offers techniques for clearing the chakras, grounding, and there is even one for helping children fall asleep. This book was worth its weight in gold when I was beginning the task of introducing meditation to my children. At just 7 and 10 years old, they both fully grasped the concept and use meditation for stress reduction. I can't say that they were ready to incorporate meditation into their daily lives as a practice which requires discipline kids this age don't have yet, but they were able to learn when they needed it as they begin to feel confident in its results. You might have fun with the activities in this book too!

So, who should meditate? Simply put, everyone. And why? Well, LIFE! Life has a way of throwing all sorts of surprises and challenges at us, and if we can meet each challenge with the resolve and confidence that we can accomplish anything, the outcome will serve us better, won't it? Just ten minutes a day can change your life profoundly. Think about how this chapter started with the biochemical explanation of something gone wrong in an autistic child's nervous system and ended with a simple solution for everyone in your life to help move that biochemical imbalance in the right direction. Knowledge is power, and the learning doesn't stop here!

---

1. C.E. Robertson, E.M. Ratai, and N. Kanwisher. *Reduced GABAergic Action in the Autistic Brain.* Harvard Society of Fellows, Harvard University, Cambridge, MA 02138, USA McGovern Institute for Brain Research, Massachusetts Institute of

Technology, Cambridge, MA 02138, USA Athinoula A. Martinos Center for Biomedical Imaging, Massachusetts General Hospital, Harvard Medical School, Charlestown, MA 02129, USA. 2016 Jan 11;26(1):80-5. doi: 10.1016/j.cub.2015.11.019. Epub 2015 Dec 17

2. C.C. Streeter, J.E. Jensen, R.M. Perlmutter, H.J. Cabral, H. Tian, D.B. Terhune, D.A. Ciraulo, P.F. Renshaw. *Yoga Asana Sessions Increase Brain GABA Levels: A Pilot Study*. The Journal of Alternative and Complementary Medicine Vol. 13, No. 4. Published Online: 28 May 2007 https://doi.org/10.1089/acm.2007.6338

12

Two steps forward, one back

THE ROAD TO RECOVERY IS A BUMPY ONE

" $\mathcal{C}$ *ourage is going from failure to failure without losing enthusiasm."*

-Winston Churchill

THE FIRST TIME I had even heard of drinking camel milk was when my uncle, who lived in Dubai at the time, sent me a brief article about how camel milk was tolerated by those who have allergies to cow's milk. It was interesting, I had never heard of camel milk dairies in the US. Later, I came across information about camel milk being used medicinally and even read a story about a family who used it to cure a severely debilitating parasitic infection. In my research, I discovered many benefits that would undoubtedly support children with Autism.

Camel milk is anti-viral and anti-bacterial, as well as being very similar to the human breastmilk, therefore it would ideally support the human immune system. In the PANDAS community, families were using something called IVIG which was the transfer of human immunoglobulin. Since camel immunoglobulins are a fraction of the size of human immunoglobulins, they are referred to as a nano-globulin, and they immediately pass into the blood stream when taken internally. You might say this is like a form of dietary IVIG.

There were too many benefits to using camel milk NOT to try it, but where on earth would I find a camel dairy?? As luck would have it, two of the very few camel dairies in the US were in my state, my very big state! My husband just happened to be going to the area where one of them was located, for work that day. To give you an idea of the serendipity of this situation, Dave probably traveled to this particular location just twice that entire year. I contacted the farmer and arranged a meeting. Dave picked up our first batch of camel milk that day! I don't believe in coincidence. The Universe at work, again.

FROM THE VERY FIRST SIP, we saw incredible, undeniable gains, including significant weight gain. Gavin had been previously diagnosed as failure to thrive and he remained at the same 27 pounds for over a year, yet within just two days of drinking camel milk by the pint, he gained two pounds, and within the next week, another pound. We were literally flabbergasted. We also saw more awareness, cognition, better speech, better executive functioning, increased humor, flat tummies for both boys (bacterial overgrowth caused chronic, visible bloating in our children) and more gains than I can even recall. We saw so many immediate gains that my best friend (who had been trialing the camel milk with her daughter as well), and I decided to start a camel milk group on Facebook called *"Healing with Camel Milk"* and ultimately acquired thousands of members from all over the world. We had guidance from the best in the industry, including an Israeli researcher who had facilitated many studies with children, using camel milk for health purposes. We had camel farmers from all over the world connecting to families through us. "Healing with Camel Milk" was connecting people with information and hope. It even attracted the interest of a grass roots film crew, the What Took You So Long Foundation, who was in the process of creating a film about camel milk for healing and had already visited 18 countries for filming. My friend and I were honored to be filmed for their documentary, "Respect the Camel Milk!"

For nine months, we gave our children camel milk daily, a pint each. When we decided to take a break from it, the only reversal of benefits we saw was a slight reduction in the weight gain they had experienced. Although camel milk held massive healing powers, it couldn't single-handedly tackle the beast that was rising in Grayson. He was thrust into the PANDAS flare of the decade due to mold exposures, both at home and at school.

THE WORD PANDAS probably conjures up thoughts of a big, fuzzy, cuddly bear, right? Cuddly and fuzzy are the last words I would use to define PANDAS. It's as much a mouthful to say Pediatric Autoimmune Neuropsychiatric Disorder Associated with Streptococcus, as it is to manage. It can also be referred to as PANS (Pediatric Acute onset Neuropsychiatric Syndrome) and the names can be used interchangeably. The reason for the updated name is because the triggers are now known to be much broader than just streptococcus, although that is one of the primary infections associated with this autoimmune disorder. In addition to streptococcal bacteria, other known infectious triggers for PANS are: Lyme and it's con-infections, clostridia, mycoplasma pneumonia, viruses like influenza, human herpesvirus 6 (HHV-6), herpes simplex virus (Type 1 and 2), parvovirus B19, coxsackievirus, Epstein–Barr virus, cytomegalovirus and candida. Non-infectious agents include certain metabolic conditions (diabetes, lupus), hormonal changes, environmental exposure to heavy metals, mold toxins, and psychological stressors.[1] There are likely many more triggers PANDAS/PANS, which have not been identified yet.

Once this disorder is triggered, (which can involve a slow or sudden onset) it can wax and wane with continued exposure to additional triggers. In affected children, the pathogen antibodies are attacking the basal ganglia of the brain typified by a common triad of symptoms: OCD, tics and rages. Some of the more common symptoms of PANDAS/PANS are easy to miscalculate as being caused by other illnesses, but when you look at the big picture and see a number of these symptoms co-existing in the same child/person, it's likely that you are looking at a case of PANDAS?PANS.

These symptoms could include, but are not limited to: obsessive-compulsive behaviors like eating disorders, fear of germs, hair pulling, and in our case, the need to control everything in his environment, motor and verbal tics (Tourette's), symptoms of hyperactivity like ADD and ADHD, learning disorders especially involving mathematics, separation anxiety, mood changes that result in sadness, irritability and emotional ups and downs, sleep disturbances, bed-wetting, urinary frequency, fine and gross motor changes resulting in visible changes in writing and drawing which waxes and wanes with the flares, and joint pains.

It's quite amazing to witness the difference in handwriting and drawing during and between these flares. When put side by side, they appear to come from a toddler and an older child. We had experienced most of the above symptoms, but it is not necessary to experience them all in order to seek the help of an educated practitioner. It is quite common to see it misdiagnosed, because this disorder is not yet widely known. You will find more alternative practitioners on board with testing for PANDAS/PANS, although there are some mainstream doctors spear-heading treatment.

It is recognized by the NIMH (the National Institute of Mental Health) and is briefly discussed on their website, although their description of the onset is quite limited and incomplete according to the real life cases I am familiar with. Many cases have a long, slow onset, with or without a known bout of strep throat or scarlet fever. Although the name suggests this is only a disorder found in children, I can personally attest to the fact that there are many adults who are also affected by this illness. Its onset is often in childhood (hence the name pediatric), but considering how common it is to misdiagnose, there are probably many adults medicating for mental disorders such as depression and OCD, who may actually have PANDAS/PANS! In fact, many of the parents who begin to look into it more for their children, discover that they once experienced many of the onset symptoms themselves at one time, perhaps as a "phase" as was once common to hear parents describe episodes involving a tic or a behavior shift. I would urge anyone dealing with depression, obsessive-compulsive disorder and/or addictions of various kinds to consider PANDAS/PANS as the possible culprit. Having personally experienced a facial tic as a child, rages after my amalgams were all put in at one office visit in high school, obsessive compulsive disorder and eventually depression, I discovered my own possible triggers.

Most conventional doctors are going to resort to medication such as prophylactic antibiotics and SSRIs (Selective Serotonin Reuptake Inhibitor) antidepressants, neither of which heal nor benefit the person long-term. Homeopathy has proven to be successful at ameliorating the symptoms, as well as healing the cause, and there are quite a few homeopaths specialized in handling PANDAS/PANS cases. Since homeopathy is a treatment that can be procured from anywhere in the world, there is no need to find someone local who is capable of handling these complex cases. The right homeopath is right at your fingertips!

GRAYSON HAD BEEN in remission from PANDAS since we found balance using herbal anti-microbials. Treatment for Autism and PANDAS are parallel in many ways, so Grayson's PANDAS went into remission temporarily by sheer coincidence because of the way we were handling his Autism. However, a new and more severe episode was triggered when he experienced exposure to mold, both at home and at school, concurrently. This served as a reminder that his health was still so fragile. More and more, we were feeling the growing pains of focusing on killing off the pathogens we felt were responsible for his episodes.

We completed an extensive remediation project at home, pulled him out of school and decided to homeschool, which was one of the absolute best decisions we have ever made for our children. He was not himself at all. His rages were out of control. He was growing bigger and the rages were becoming just as hefty. At seven years old, he was more aware of his imbalances too. He was no longer the toddler who would respond to simple distraction, he was fully immersed in his anger, and equally as consumed by his remorse.

———

HIS VOICE SLICED through the silence, howling, this time over having to come in from playing outside. My stomach ached with emotions ranging from downright frustration to sadness and discouragement. I didn't know what to do for him.

"*Grayson,*" I called up to him while listening to things clattering and pounding in his room. It felt like the ceiling might come down. "What IS he doing?" I thought to myself. As I entered his bedroom, which had become a battleground, he threw himself defiantly on his bed, arms crossed, face firm, chin jutting out away from my solemn stare. It was obvious he wasn't prepared to talk to me yet. So I just sat there, looking at him in silence, processing this scene. His brother peeking into the room broke the silence.

"*Gavin, can you please give us a few minutes?*" I said, wishing Dave were home from his trip to help me. I knew Gavin needed comforting too, as these outbursts were unsettling and affected the whole family.

With that, Grayson broke down, arms still crossed in defiance, glancing down at his bedspread, "*I don't know what is wrong with me, I get so angry and I can't control it when it starts. I'm sorry....do you forgive me?*" I immediately scooped his sobbing body into mine and sobbed with him...for him. At least he now allowed me to comfort him.

HE HAD BEEN angry so often. I was heartbroken over his inability to control his own actions and that he had to feel such painful remorse, yet exhausted with these conversations. He didn't deserve this. He was a child, and his life should be full of excitement and wonder, not riddled with inner pain, self-doubt and anger. We went into yet another discussion about using deep breaths to calm down and using our words to express feelings before it gets out of control. The truth is, when he was unwell, he was incapable of stopping the flow of emotions. It was like a damn broke in his mind, and once he was triggered, the anger was intractable. Then we started the same cycle of apologies and discussions over again. I was, however, grateful to see that he was experiencing remorse on a more consistent basis. Remorse is something we rarely saw when he was fitting into the Autism diagnosis. Although Autism had been replaced by the monster we called PANDAS/PANS, I had to consciously remind myself to focus on the positive, even if these details felt few and far between.

WE HAD GONE from throwing everything but the kitchen sink at him, to feeling lost and empty with our new desire to back down from the growing list of supplements and antimicrobials. It just didn't feel right to keep feeding our kids synthetic supplements. With each passing pill, and there were many, I felt my heart skip a beat. It was time to follow my instincts more. Moving from a rigid protocol to....who knows? After years of feeling settled into a plan that held so much hope for us, it was confusing and disheartening. As we watched Grayson's ability to function normally decrease even with the increasing doses of natural antimicrobials, we knew we had to do something different. This just wasn't cutting it any longer. Gripping fear was beginning to seep in.

IN A BITTERSWEET EXPERIENCE of observing Grayson as he read to me while struggling with debilitating tics that swept over his face every few minutes. I had a burning desire to kick this illness you-know-where. I couldn't make out if these were still tics (they tended to shift pretty regularly) or if he was experiencing seizures. Grayson's tics had a rotational quality about them. He shifted in and out of various verbal and physical tics over the years, some of which even looked like something else entirely. His newest tic caused his eyes to flutter up and over to one side hard, where he would stare for a few seconds at a time. They were so troublesome that I secretly recorded him and sent it to our MD/homeopath who calmed my nerves by confirming that they were in fact tics, not seizures (which are actually a common condition to co-exist with PANS). Although I was grateful they weren't seizures, I was completely sick to my stomach and consumed with a feeling of failure, yet again. I couldn't let this illness take us down, I wouldn't allow it. It was time to cultivate a stronger belief system.

---

1. https://www.thescienceofpsychotherapy.com/understanding-pans-pandas/

13

Overflowing buckets

MAKING SENSE OF THE ROLE TOXINS PLAY
IN CHRONIC ILLNESS

"*A wareness is the greatest agent for change.*"

-Eckhart Tolle

Now THAT YOU have seen just from our experience how many things can contribute to the complex threads in the tapestry of Autism and PANDAS/PANS, I'd like to share a visual with you which may help in your quest for recovery. It can feel so overwhelming to consider all the possible causes that contribute to Autism and PANDAS/PANS. This visual will highlight an overall picture of what is going on with our kids that will make this journey almost appear manageable, because it simplifies the mass of information into one story per child.

Imagine a bucket. Yup, just a good old fashioned bucket that you would fill with soapy water to wash your car. Instead of filling it with water, imagine this bucket as your child's immune system which comes predisposed genetically and its contents are the triggers and toxins that overwhelm your child's immune system.

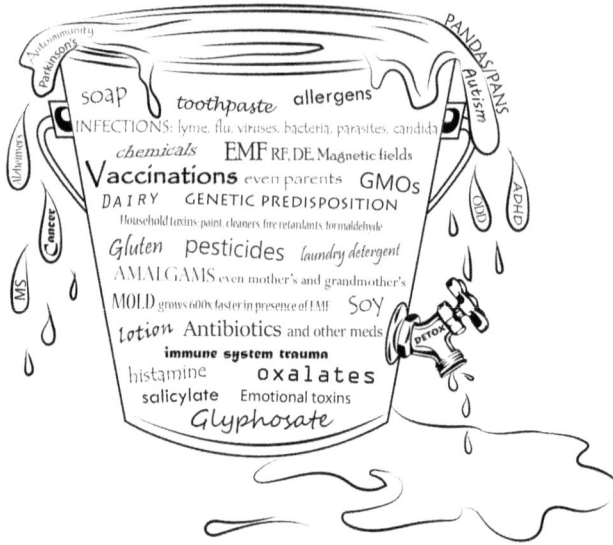

As each toxin enters your child's bucket, it fills the bucket a little more each time, or sometimes a lot, depending on the impact of each trigger on your child's immune system. For example, smelling diesel fumes might only increase the contents of the bucket slightly, while a vaccination could fill a quarter or even half of the bucket all at once. For another child, it might be the complete opposite. It all depends on the genetic makeup of the child and what they are predisposed to. Also understand that children are no longer born with empty buckets, some are even already full upon entering this world. If the child has an effective detoxification system, most of these things will filter out faster than they build up, whereas children with slower detoxification pathways will hold onto these toxins, filling up the bucket faster than others. Once their bucket reaches its capacity, there is nowhere for the contents to go so they must over-flow and spill out - it's this overflow that represents a child's Autism/PANDAS/PANS, or other chronic conditions. There was a time, not too long ago, when it took an entire lifetime to fill up these buckets, which would result in dementia, arthritis, cancer, slower mental capacities, etc., but now we are seeing children with some of the same diseases that were previously only experienced by the elderly.

So, imagine this invisible bucket which fills up with each insult, and in a matter of time, the bucket becomes full, eventually overflowing to create the symptoms we refer to as Autism and PANDAS/PANS. For one child, the final insult might be their vaccinations, for another it might be a virus, and for yet another it could be mold or a troubling food they are eating on a regular basis. Even emotional toxins will add to their buckets and can sometimes be overwhelming enough to be the icing on the cake...or the water overflowing the bucket.

THERE ARE two key components to maintaining your child's bucket. First, you must determine what toxins are contributing to their bucket accumulation. Is it antimony from their mattresses and pajamas? Could it be the emotional pressure from a teacher or parent to behave more maturely when their development simply prevents it? Is it the gluten, dairy and soy in their diets? Maybe they used soy formula as an infant, or does it extend further into their diets with the accumulation of oxalates or salicylates? Could it be the mold they are encountering at school or the constant strep infections? You get the picture.

There may be many triggers, but anything that changes their disposition or behaviors should absolutely be tagged as problematic, no matter how much you want to deny it. I know you will...we did. It's a natural defense mechanism, but this will only get in the way of your recovery if you allow it to continue.

Sometimes testing can help you identify potential sources of trouble since it can be hard to decipher what is involved in filling your child's bucket. It's not always black and white.

For us, fecal testing with unconventional labs was pivotal in identifying microbes that were overgrown and IgG food panels helped us navigate the food triggers, while organic acid testing uncovered neurotransmitter imbalances and gene testing shed light on why that might be happening. It all came down to our detox pathways in the end, but knowing these things was confirming and sometimes shocking, but empowering too. It gave me direction and insight I needed to continue on the path, as I was learning what to prioritize.

Some of these things can be a challenge to manage, which brings me to key component number two: managing the bucket to prevent overflow. This means stepping in and finding solutions to any of the things that are triggering your child in any way. Take it one step at a time. Don't look ahead, and definitely don't look back, only focus on what you can handle today. If you just witnessed your child have a tantrum, because s/he ate something with honey in it, start there. Removing the honey would be the first step, taking it deeper would be to see if honey is one of the many high salicylate foods to cause a problem. Try to broaden the picture a little bit starting with the honey. Does s/he also react to other high salicylate foods on the list like coconut, or is it just the honey? Once you've removed the honey, watch for other triggers and deal with them when you can. For example, doing a hair mineral analysis might uncover an antimony toxicity which requires a major overhaul in the house, starting with the costly job of replacing mattresses and carpeting, in which case you may have to put those items on the back burner until you can prioritize them. In the meantime, do what you can to reduce antimony in smaller ways, like avoiding pajamas with fire retardant. Every little bit counts, every little bit is part of the bucket overflow. The larger things will most likely be a bigger chunk of the recovery and will need to be dealt with at some time, somehow, but don't stress if you can't deal with it now. Instead, put a plan in place to help you feel like you ARE addressing it. Maybe a savings plan to pay for a new mattress is enough to put this concern to the side for now.

Stressing about it will only add to your own bucket. So approach each step with the attitude that you will do what you can, when you can. Take on the more manageable tasks first and you will be amazed at how things just seem to smooth over in time.

WHEN I WAS NURSING Gavin who is three years younger than Grayson, I discovered that my amalgams had contributed to

Grayson's bucket toxins and that they might have been a very large part of his overflow. You can imagine the distress I felt initially when I realized that I was poisoning my baby with mercury every time I nursed him. What an oxymoron, the milk he was supposed to be nourished by was literally poisoning him with heavy metals every day, which could have easily made me feel like it was my fault that I was poisoning him. I would literally sob over it as I nursed him. I couldn't help but wonder if I was going to contribute to a regression into Autism for him as well. I also knew that breastmilk was a healthier food than formula and he wanted to nurse, unlike Grayson who fought me and weaned himself at three months old. I welcomed this bond, I wanted to nourish his body with this custom supply of food that was designed just for him.

So I stopped crying, I held him close, I stayed focused on the very moment I was experiencing with my baby. I had to put my fears away temporarily, because I knew that messing with my amalgams in any way while he was still nursing was like releasing a weapon of mass destruction into his little body. Doing my best in that moment meant continuing to nurse him without stressing us both out. I knew I had to address the amalgams for my own health, but I also knew it was too late to replace them in order to prevent toxicity in my baby. It would make no sense to dwell on this, so I continued nursing and reminded myself that I would do what I could, when I could.

Do what you can, remove the problematic foods, stop the vaccinations, replace your cleaning and personal care products with safer options, invest in the Dirty Dozen organic foods (strawberries, spinach, kale, nectarines, apples, grapes, peaches, cherries, pears, tomatoes, celery and potatoes) and don't worry so much about the Clean Fifteen (avocado, sweet corn, pineapples, frozen sweet peas, onions, papayas, eggplants, kiwis, cabbage, cauliflower, cantaloupes, broccoli, mushrooms and honeydew) if you can't afford a full organic diet. Maybe you need a new perspective on what is important in that moment, like I did, and use supplements, probiotics, herbals and/or homeopathy to strengthen their immune system, encourage gentle detox, and prevent microbial overgrowth and illness.

EVERY LITTLE IMPROVEMENT is akin to opening the spigot at the bottom of the bucket just a little bit more and will contribute to draining out the accumulation over time. When you are able to maintain your child's bucket, you will begin to see patterns of health and illness emerge within your control. This can be eye opening and empowering at the same time. It will motivate you further, and the reward for your hard work makes it all worth it. It is life changing! Your child's PANDAS/PANS can go into remission and your child's Autism symptoms can reduce or even dissolve entirely as you find the right combination of solutions for maintaining their bucket. It did for us!

With this in mind, it also means that in many situations, you (and your child as s/he grows older) will always need to keep your bucket maintained, because of its tendency to fill up faster than the average person. They likely have genetic mutations contributing to their bucket-filling predisposition so there will be a lifetime of monitoring required to maintain health. There will be times when a particular trigger or a set of triggers causes what appears to be regression or a resurgence of symptoms. Don't worry, over time you will also realize what it takes to regain health again. Each experience will help you build your toolbox. Sometimes it's as simple as cutting back on a food you may have reintroduced as part of a challenge, or it may require a complete overhaul and restructuring of your perspective, but if you keep your focus on what has recently changed, you are more likely to recover from the blip faster. And be prepared for hormonal disruptions, they can throw parents for a loop when they aren't expecting it!

THE KEY to the proverbial "finish line" that I used to envision begins right here. This is it!! Once you have decoded your child's triggers and you continue to identify items that add to the bucket, and more importantly how to prevent them from filling up too fast, you have begun to unlock the key to your child's puzzle. From here on out, your job (and your child's if they go on to live independently) is to maintain their buckets just like you maintain your house, regular house cleaning a little at a time goes a long way. It's essential to their continued health.

Be prepared to discover that the apple doesn't fall far from the tree, if you haven't already. As you are uncovering your child's triggers, you may also uncover your own. Embrace this process, as it may provide the key to your own chronic ailments. It will most certainly aid in prevention as well.

Navigating this journey added to my toolbox, allowing me to find additional solutions to the many challenges we were being faced with. Just knowing that I needed to manage my boys' buckets (and my own) wasn't enough, I had to trudge around in the myriad of options out there. Which ones were right for us, and which are right for you? The only way to know is to try them on for size and place them into the helpful or disastrous files for future reference. The rest of my journey will explain how I came to trust myself more.

14

The habit of fear

HOW CONDITIONING CONTROLS OUR AUTOMATIC RESPONSE TO THE ENVIRONMENT

"*We can never obtain peace in the outer world until we make peace within ourselves.*"

-*Dalai Lama*

FEAR AS A HABIT means the subconscious has defaulted to a pattern of negative thinking in response to the environment. How does the habit of fear develop? It can be slow and insidious or it can come on suddenly and violently. It just depends on the personal experience that defines your fear(s). Many parents of special needs children would agree that they suffer from some form of PTSD (Post-traumatic stress disorder). It's inevitable for the caregivers of someone suffering with chronic illness of an emotional nature. The physical and emotional can become directly connected with each new trauma, although when we dig deeper we will often find a history associated with certain triggers. Stories from the past are replayed when triggers set the stage for fear to surface.

Everything has a cause, an origin, a place where the "thing" has it's beginning. We aren't always privy to this magical point of origin when contemplating a cure to an illness, but think of how easy healing would be, if we were consciously connected to this place and time. Perhaps we could even just rewind back through it and eliminate the "thing" causing us pain. Unfortunately, it's not that simple. We struggle with the cause of dis-ease, we focus on the disease, the pain, the symptoms, and in fact, this is the very foundation of medical and scientific research. We wonder, why did he get cancer? How did she end up with multiple sclerosis? And as many of you reading this have probably thought, why did my child win the Autism lottery? If we knew, could we reverse it, or even better, prevent it to begin with? I believe that the cause of an illness is not necessarily unique to the illness any more than a cause can induce the same symptoms in every person who has it. Let me explain myself.

Tracing backwards, the cause is dependent on the person's miasms (which are a person's inherent susceptibilities and predispositions), according to a combination of their genetic components, emotional experiences and environmental exposures, potentially stemming back long before the symptoms surfaced in the physical body, possibly even before birth, as miasms are generational. Then we have triggers which too often become entangled and confused with the cause of the "thing." They are, however, different.

A trigger for asthma is often intense activity, but it is not the CAUSE for the asthma. The trigger activates the red flag, a symptom, but it has very little to do with the origin of the dis-ease state. Herein lies the very disconnect in conventional treatment options. The origin of any dis-ease state is much deeper than its symptoms. Can we treat the results of the trigger? Sure. This is, in effect, the basis of most allopathic medicine. We can swallow a pain reliever for a headache, but if the cause of the headache is an environmental allergy or a food sensitivity, that pain reliever is doing absolutely nothing to address the cause, and the episode is likely to repeat itself again and again. The problem is that conventional medicine often aims at anti-symptom, stop the red flag from waving you down, so you think you are in the clear. Treating the symptom is not the same as treating the cause.

Imagine if you took your car to the mechanic because the "check engine" indicator was on and your mechanic disconnected the power to the check engine light and sent you on your way. No light, no problem, right? Wrong. Most conventional medicine is palliative in nature and rarely addresses the cause. Palliative care is the equivalence of disconnecting the power to the check engine light. We should be asking ourselves WHY does the child have asthma to begin with, what caused it in the first place? When we ignore the cause and repeatedly treat the symptoms, we are suppressing the body's innate healing response. Symptoms are actually a sign that the body is attempting to heal itself! A fever is designed to kill off a pathogen, bleeding cleans out the wound, inflammation introduces the appropriate cells to the injured site. When we stop these processes from occurring, we are suppressing the natural healing of the body.

Suppression pushes the action inward, where it may possibly cause more damage, long- term. True recovery from dis-ease must occur in layers and may unleash multiple trigger/symptom patterns from the past. As our life force strengthens, it will naturally throw off the energy of these old vibrations which are still imprinted in our bodies. On the physical level, healing liberates toxins that were once stored in our tissues, which releases the toxins into the bloodstream, causing old symptoms to return. It is actually a sign of healing (also known as a "healing crisis" or in homeopathy, referred to as "rewind") to see the temporary return of old symptoms, both physical and emotional. In the allopathic model, the return of old symptoms elicits fear. It brings on negative thought patterns and this drives the need to palliate. It's an engrained pattern of conditioning that we get subconsciously trapped into.

When I was a bystander of the Biomedical approach to healing Grayson, I was hypersensitive to every "symptom" he expressed. While on one hand, I could argue that this activated a response that led me to address the issue, it actually just kept me in a constant state of fight or flight. I was chasing the symptoms, and suppressing them left and right. I was led to believe that I was doing the right thing because he always responded favorably to my methods of suppression. If that isn't the ultimate oxymoron right there...

The problem was that the pattern continued to repeat itself, because true healing hadn't taken place. I was suppressing symptoms so rather than liberating toxins and eliminating the suppression of biomedicine was encouraging the body to store toxins. I spent years wanting, expecting everything to make perfect sense, for there to be this linear path to recovery where all the details would fall neatly into their right places logically. I expected treatment to heal the proposed symptoms without failure. Thankfully, I eventually recognized the pattern and pulled us out of its grip, but obviously that didn't happen overnight.

FOR ME, despair crept into my bones slowly and silently. I was oblivious. I didn't see the shadow behind me growing larger and more powerful. I was too focused on the treacherous path before me. I was too busy clearing the way through an overgrown forest of foreign challenges, one after the other. My adrenaline didn't slow down enough for me to pause and take it all in. I had never thought we wouldn't win this battle, but deep down inside, the seed of fear had somehow already been planted...and it was taking root.

This was all new to me. I had never experienced illness like this. I had to forge my way alone. No family members or friends to relate to, and none to relate to me. It was a lonely corner to be in. I yearned for compassion, understanding and support. Unfortunately, no one in my family understood what we were going through, nor did I share much. On one hand, I resented their lack of interest, and on the other hand, I didn't want our child to be harshly judged, so we kept to ourselves. This balance was a double-edged sword. Fear had crept in.

My response to the kids began to change, a new tic would throw me off kilter for days, a tantrum would send me into my own world where I could hide my emotions, my patience grew thinner, my sleep became shallower and I was feeling frail myself. I began having thoughts that we couldn't go on like this, but what could give? What room was there for anything to change? We weren't living this way because we wanted to, it felt like we HAD to. I felt like I was traveling through an endless dark tunnel. Where was the light, isn't there always light at the end of the tunnel?

We were so engulfed in the life we had created, and we were in over our heads. I couldn't see life the same way most people did anymore. Chronic illness changes you in ways you can't imagine. I had a new perspective of the world around us and it wasn't a pretty one. Hopelessness lurked around every corner. Carnivals were too loud and frightening for Grayson, walking around a festival or park was too physically exhausting for him, and if it was summer, it was too hot for him and he would become itchy, rashy and irritable. These were all signs that his mitochondria were failing at their duty to provide his body with energy. Preparing for a full day out became too exhausting!

It wasn't until we were really coming out of the storm that I turned around and saw it on my tail. RIGHT on my tail! Fear! I had opened the front door and let the beast right in my home. How did that happen? When did that happen?

This habit of fear grabbed a hold of us and wouldn't let go easily. I can recall days when I was consciously teaching myself to be less reactive, where I would notice my old instincts trying to kick in, I would watch them trying to take over, as I struggled to remain calm. It was the habit of fear, driving my actions and words.

Thinking back to one of our more fear-driven experiences when Grayson was a toddler...

Glancing at the clock across the room, I swallow hard and my eyes immediately dart to meet Dave's, I could see that he instantly knew what this look meant. We had an unspoken communication that many parents with a high needs child can relate to. He shifted uneasily in his seat at the table, as my nerves began to fray. It was nearing 6:30 pm. We were barely finished with dinner. I could see him thoughtfully processing how we would gracefully end our visit even though no one had even begun to open their Christmas gifts yet. We knew we would have to cut yet another family gathering short. The witching hour was right around the corner and we were cutting it really close.

Although Grayson was happily enjoying the company of his cousins now, we both knew that like the flip of a switch, at just the right time, he would no longer be this calm, beaming little boy representing the wonder of Christmas cheer. I wanted nothing more than to protect this innocent image of our precious boy. The beautiful child sitting beside me appeared to exhibit patience, confidence and pure joy. This was how I wanted him to remain in everyone's eyes. To let people in, meant allowing this image to be shattered with the harsh truth of what lies on the other side of the wall that protected us from judgement. The reality of what we were going through could be confusing, depressing and sometimes downright terrifying. I recognized that this was hard to understand for those on the outside, which perpetuated the isolation we lived in. Protecting our loved ones from this reality meant putting on a mask of courage and poise while going through the motions of a lifestyle that was still new even to us, as first time parents of a child with an invisibly debilitating condition. We knew what we had to do. We'd been through it too many times. If Grayson wasn't in his bed by 7pm sharp, the night would be long and painful for everyone. It wouldn't be fair to Grayson. If we pushed him to the brink of tolerance, he suffered tremendously, and so did we.

Since Grayson had been a baby, overstimulation and staying awake until he got overtired opened the doorway to anxiety, OCD, and tears, lots of tears. Suddenly everything that had ever disturbed him was magnified a hundred times during the night hours, and like Cinderella's midnight chariot, poof, Grayson's cortisol levels would soar, driving him (and us) to madness. No amount of soothing, bribing or rationalizing could calm him when he reached this state. He would wake no less than five times at night, stumbling into our room in a frenzy, needing help to settle back down enough to fall asleep. To make matters worse, once we had triggered even just one night of this, it would literally take days to get him back on schedule. We endured days of this overtired, unreasonable, oversensitive state, with all of our sleep disturbed. This sort of disruption trickled into the daytime with increased sensitivities and tantrums over any hiccup in his expectations. His central nervous system couldn't handle the upset of even one night of schedule disturbance. We all suffered. My ability to balance nursing Gavin a couple of times at night, with the random wake up calls from Grayson who couldn't settle back to sleep was compounded by Dave's business travel, which was also unpredictable. We had to balance the consequences of our choices against our need for calm, peace and sleep!

We knew that we would inevitably disappoint family who couldn't quite understand how this happy toddler, who was currently smiling and cooperating, would require such drastic measures as cutting a holiday celebration short. But if we didn't leave with plenty of time to get him home BEFORE his bedtime, everything would spiral out of control quickly. How do you explain such drama to people you love, who would most likely see this as a discipline issue, rather than what it really was...Autism and PANDAS. This was disappointment on a different level. We were regularly stuck with decisions that would hurt someone, in order to keep some sense of normalcy in our day to day lives. No one could quite understand what we were going through, hence the divide.

The guilt was already building, and we knew that the instant one of us made the first move to leave, all eyes would be on us. Painfully, every second felt like an eternity, but I waited for Dave to make that first move. I noticed I was holding my breath. But why? Why must we fear the choices we need to make for our family's best interest? He's standing, I can see the agony on his face, I released my breath. The guilt, our own fear, coupled with knowing we've let those we love down. It stings. Be strong. Taking another deep breath, I stood and attempted to make eye contact with Grayson, who clearly was not ready to go either. I sensed the confusion in the air.

"We haven't even opened presents yet?" it stung like a knife to the heart.

"We'll have to take them with us, we have to get the boys to bed. Grayson needs a lot of down time before he can fall asleep," I mustered up in an attempt to explain our need to leave early, again, only serving to create a greater divide.

Awkward silence

I KNEW what they were thinking, or at least I thought I did. Either way, it was not comfortable for anyone. So we packed up in silence and said our disappointed goodbyes with forced smiles on our faces, and took the wrapped gifts with us. And as if we didn't know why we were doing this, both Dave and I erupted in over the top explanation when we reached the privacy of our car. We were trying to convince ourselves that this was the right thing to do. We already KNEW it was the right thing to do, for Grayson, for all of us. No one in our immediate family knew what it was like to live on the eggshells, no the landmines of Autism....when there was an explosion, we were all hit by the shrapnel. But we explained ourselves silly anyway, in an attempt to ease the pain of having to disappoint people we love - in order to protect someone we love. Our life required us to get tough, to re-write our thought patterns and old habits, but it wasn't easy.

IN ORDER TO ACCEPT CHANGE, we must be willing to re-write the past. Letting go and trusting is a huge part of this process. Many don't even know they are holding onto old stories, they only recognize the familiar and feared outcome. We need to face our past head-on and reorganize our thoughts. In hindsight, I see now that breaking down the walls of fear requires miracles and we must believe in these miracles for them to find their place in our lives. I was determined to change these habits. Throughout the course of our recovery, I could feel us flow in and out of our old habits as we attempted to create new ones. It takes a conscious effort and a lot of dedication to make permanent change, but I was determined!

The painful truth is that fear can only take hold if you allow it. The evolution of illness has two paths; a choose-your-own-adventure series, if you will. Down one path, you can take in each experience and patiently explore it, and allow it to unfold before you and be willing to find the lesson in it. This is where the learning happens, where we find our purpose. Down the other path, you can give strength and power to fear, and you can become reactive and attached to an outcome, in which case, there is always going to be pain. This would become my lesson as we navigated through life with chronic illness.

15

Onward and upward

A SHIFT IN THE HEALING PARADIGM TURNS UP SOIL-BASED ORGANISMS

"It is only through labor and painful effort, by grim energy and resolute courage, that we move on to better things."

-Theodore Roosevelt

GRAYSON'S PANDAS symptoms had us all on edge. It was time for change, so I went back into research mode and with the idea that I didn't want to kill off any more beneficial bacteria (or encourage the overgrowth of pathogenic bacteria). I focused my research on building up the gut terrain and came across soil based organisms (SBOs), which are a form of probiotic. Probiotics are supplemental good bacteria, and the word probiotic actually means "for life." They appeared almost miraculous. I did more research every day, well into the nights. I felt like I was on to something, something really big, but I couldn't find other Autism/PANDAS families using SBOs. So, I dug a bit deeper, read studies, read articles about their safety and their risks, listened to presentations from doctors who sang their praises and when I learned that they would improve digestion, decrease toxic overload, as well as fight off all non-beneficial microbes, INCLUDING MOLD, I was sold.

I was very particular about the brand though, because many brands had questionable ingredients added to them. I wanted a good, soil-based probiotic, nothing added. I avoided strep thermophilus because of the cross reactivity experienced in kids with PANDAS, barley grass, as well as maltodextrin which is a corn-based ingredient, and likely to be GMO (genetically modified organism) too.

I settled on a brand, contacted the Vice President with my many questions and then moved on it. We had a new, promising plan. I was beyond excited at this point, and with good reason. I immediately dropped all antimicrobials. I wanted to really give the probiotics a shot at success. I didn't want to interfere with products that might potentially kill them. So risking regression, we jumped in head first.

I was on the phone with the Vice President a few times a week, looking for reassurance that we were seeing progress, because without the antimicrobials, it felt like we were seeing a lot of what felt like regression. I was teetering on panic most days. But I had hope and faith, and the Vice President was reassuring me every step of the way. It would work, it WILL work! After a few months of managing the s-l-o-w and painful increase of their doses, we reached a plateau and low and behold, we had flat bellies, calm children, and we had major, major improvement!! All this without the antimicrobials. I still couldn't believe that we were maintaining with nothing but probiotics! I was ecstatic and had to scream it from mountaintops! So in my usual way, I wrote about them in my blog and I shared with everyone and anyone who seemed like they could benefit from them.

Here is a small portion of my praise of the SBOs from my blog:

"In one word....UNBELIEVABLE!! We did something completely radical and dropped ALL of the natural antimicrobials to give this probiotic a fair shot at combating the dysbiosis. I must admit, it was scary while we were going through it, because I didn't know half the time if we were seeing die-off or

overgrowth, since we were using nothing else. We continued to work our 6 year old up to 6 capsules a day and our 3 year old somewhere between 3 and 4. After only one and a half months on the product, I am ecstatic to report that we have an OAT (organic acid test) and two stool tests (these were only done for Gavin so far) to confirm that we are completely in control of the dysbiosis!! Grayson's previous OAT had a level of 413 for HPHPA (clostridia) which we battled for a good year with natural antimicrobials, this new test result is....DRUM ROLL PLEASE...26!!! And yeast markers are totally normal, all around. Gavin had slightly higher numbers, but remember that we only just recently got him up to 3 capsules. My guess is that the dose is directly correlated with the results, because a friend who also has a daughter who just recently (just two months ago) had a level of 393 for Clostridia and confirmed Candida Krusei, just resulted in 22 for the HPHPA and normal levels of yeast, and NO Candida Krusei to speak of, as well!! She was also on 6 capsules."

So, now we had the amazing progress from using the soil-based organisms, but we wanted deeper healing. It wasn't enough to just maintain the pathogenic overgrowth. If we wanted the pathogenic overgrowth to cease, we had to aim for the root cause and heal that. The SBOs were effectively addressing the physical dysbiosis, now it was time to super-charge healing by combining the SBOs with homeopathy.

16

Homeopathy revisited

"*If at first you don't succeed, try, try again.*"

-William Edward Hickson

We had already been working with a classical homeopath for a year and a half, and although we experienced an immediate response to his constitutional remedy, the improvements fizzled.

I loved homeopathy and always had faith in its abilities (it had proven to be amazing when used acutely, as well as in helping me get off of SSRIs), but after a year and a half on the same remedy, we just weren't seeing the additional progress we wanted or expected. His PANDAS/PANS symptoms were progressively getting worse and his homeopath held firm with his constitutional remedy. It had its place in our journey and the gains remained, but it was feeling like it was time to move on. I found myself questioning the one-remedy approach, I was feeling as though we needed more remedies to address multiple layers of healing.

Through genetic testing, we had learned about our methylation pathways and how genetic mutations can block detox, if they are being expressed. Methylation is the process of taking a single carbon and three hydrogens, known as a "methyl group," and applying it to multiple functions in the body. Methylation impacts detoxification, neurotransmitter production, histamine metabolism, estrogen metabolism, DNA production, liver health, eye health, turning genes on and off, fighting infections, fat metabolism and cellular energy. When methylation is impaired, a wide variety of symptoms can ensue. It is common for practitioners to recommend supplements according to the combination of SNPs (single nucleotide polymorphisms) found in the genetic testing of the methylation pathways and their coordinating symptoms. We attempted to incorporate the recommended supplements into our routine, but we all actually felt worse and were ultimately left with the feeling that such extreme supplementation was intended to "bypass" gene mutations rather than encouraging the body to change the expression of those genes. They were just another temporary bandaid. I didn't want to just bypass gene mutations, I wanted to turn their expression off (or on, depending on the gene involved). As luck would have it, an article caught my eye about a study that proved homeopathy has the power to change gene expression so I chose to research methods of opening these pathways with homeopathy. This is when Homotoxicology hit my radar.

HOMOTOXICOLOGY IS a form of healing based on homeopathy, but with a very specific purpose of opening detox pathways. It was created by German doctor Hans-Heinrich Reckeweg (1905-1985), drawing on his combined knowledge of homeopathy and herbal medicine. His focus was on creating function-based medicines (with a combined mixture of potencies in each remedy, also known as homaccords) aimed at supporting and draining organs which would ultimately open up blockages. These remedies stimulate the metabolism and tone up the immune system and organs. A combination of homeopathic nosodes, homeopathic sarcodes, vitamins and herbs (we chose not to use the herbs, because of the oxalate and salicylate sensitivities with Gavin) are used to encourage the body systems to act in harmony. Reckeweg discovered phases of toxin progression which systematically ties in with degeneration and disease. The end phase, if not addressed, can result in malignancy. In each of these phases, certain remedies are used to target the reversal of the damage occurring, and in turn, open up the detox pathways associated with that phase.

Our homotoxicologist used a biofeedback machine to test their meridians energetically. It was love at first sight! It reminded me of how many times I had said, "I wish I could just plug my kids into a machine like the one you plug a car into for diagnostics!" Well, now you can!! It was able to identify deficiencies, toxicities, pathogens, allergies, if chosen remedies resonated with the kids, and SO much more. I was hooked. In homotoxicology, there is a specific process for testing and treating, so we didn't necessarily get to learn all of those things about our children, but just knowing it was an option had me drooling. This would later drive my desire to own a similar machine.

We had a few appointments with our homotoxicologist, and our kids were testing on the practitioner's biofeedback machine very well right from the beginning. In fact, she told us that their testing looked as good as many of her clients who had been treated by her for over a year. We had done so much work already, but we knew there was more to be done. So even though her testing looked encouraging, it was purely focused on the physical aspect of illness. Although we only used it for about six months, I feel that this modality served to teach us that we could rely on homeopathic remedies without all the supplements, leading to the removal of many unnecessary supplements from our long list.

We really simplified things during this phase of healing. It felt great to only need to give a few remedies and supplements a day. I knew deep down that it was more than just the physical body that needed our focus though. I kept coming back to this, thinking healing must move beyond the physical body. Our kids needed to heal the damage from generational dis-ease. It began to feel like we were jumping from treatment to treatment, focused on just the physical, looking for the shoe that fit perfectly. I continued to follow my gut.

Through networking with other parents in the ASD and PANDAS/PANS communities, a homeopathic college was recommended to us for treatment. I was eager to let someone else handle our healing at a deeper level. Students took on cases as part of their training and I was hearing incredible healing stories from their clients. We thought we would give it a try. It was affordable and allowed us to treat the whole family at once. We continued to use the knowledge and remedies gained through our experiences with Homotoxicology, to work on organ drainage, while digging deeper to clear old "toxins."

WE BEGAN what would be an adventurous eight-month journey with a student homeopath. It was their motto to treat the whole family in order to heal the children, because (as I had also been discovering in my own reading) the family unit holds its own vibration, and this can be healthy or unhealthy depending on the patterns we are perpetuating. We can carry on these vibrational patterns from parents, grandparents and so forth, we can also create them within our own life experiences, adding to the muddied mixtures. It's as if we live in our own little vibrational bubble, intimately connected to our immediate family.

Think about it this way: if your partner comes home in a funk from something that happened at work, it quickly travels through all of the family members, unless there is one who is stronger than these vibrations and can spin it into a positive experience. When our family lacks that strong vibrational presence, one bad mood in the house can bring everyone down. And what about when you walk into a room where two people have just been arguing, you can FEEL the charge, the tension in the air is thick enough to sense. This is vibratory. You are walking into an environment where the frequencies are so different from yours in that moment, that you sense the shift, as if it were a change in temperature. And alternately, think about entering a space where everyone is lifted and joyous….a concert for instance. Music raises the vibration in the space around you, everyone is excited and enjoying themselves, you can FEEL it! These vibrations move you in the direction the vibrations are headed.

TREATMENT of our entire family was pivotal for our children, but it also created a place for me to see my role in the whole, like the compartmentalized organs in conventional medicine. I am part of the whole, my husband is part of the whole, each child is part of the same whole. I was not exempt from the effects of Autism and PANDAS/PANS in our home. None of us were. Caring for those with chronic illness effects the entire family. Siblings have to make compromises just like parents. No one is exempt. I can't stress this enough, a family is a holistic system that relies on one another to function as a whole. All family members should heal alongside the affected child. We were all affected somehow: genetically, environmentally, emotionally, and we are saturated in each other's emotions and surroundings. Am I Autistic? No, but just because we don't have Autism or PANDAS/PANS doesn't mean we are perfectly healthy either. Everyone can stand to improve their health on some level. I'm sure you can come up with something you would like to see improve. The family bubble, as I like to refer to it, also affects us all. We are all connected.

Healing together catapults healing for the effected family member, as well. It is incredible to experience the shift from "fixing" a child, to healing with a child.

It's easy to forget that our homes carry our accumulated vibration as a whole. The many exposures we have on a daily basis determine whether our vibration resonates at a higher or lower frequency. Unhealthy foods, toxins, chemicals, molds, pesticides, negative relationships, illnesses, bad moods, bad habits, stress…all carry low vibrations.

Alternatively, healthy fresh organic foods, good moods, wellness, uplifting relationships, exercise, inspiring music and anything that creates a peaceful environment will create higher vibrations. Do you tend to see the full side of the glass or the empty side of that same glass when you deal with life's challenges? Often this isn't even a conscious choice, we are programmed to respond according to pathways of reasoning that develop in early childhood, based on our surroundings. Our instinctual reaction to circumstances is well rooted and you may not even realize how you view things. I know I didn't, not until I was forced to look hard at myself as a contributor to our family energy bubble. I always thought Dave and I were calm, positive people. We rarely argued, we loved each other deeply, we were willing to do anything for another person who was in need or required help, but when I pulled out the introspection spectacles, I saw a different side of myself, one that would need attention. Treatment for the whole family is exactly what I felt drawn to, this would be our magic!

OUR HOMEOPATHIC ITINERARY consisted of remedies to support organs, remedies to clear the energy of old toxins like vaccines, medication and even supplements that were used extensively all while working with additional remedies to restore health in the physical, mental, emotional and the spiritual planes. We were seeing improvement fast. Grayson's tics were still prevalent throughout this entire process though. It was as if nothing could break through the barrier. We saw so much progress with each one of us that we held onto hope with every homeopathic pellet we put onto his tongue. Each pellet with its own story to share with us, each with its own outcome…*"Would it be THIS one?" "Is THIS the magic pellet?" "Will today be THE day?"* The hope was palpable and the progress was so fruitful in every other way that we didn't stress much over the details, we knew it would just be a matter of time. Gavin's edginess softened, Grayson's recent increase in OCD and rages were gone, dare I say it, life felt normal again!

Detox was real, and in hindsight, it was incredibly insightful. As we saw over the previous four years, as long as we kept the candida under control, we didn't see Grayson's sound defensiveness kick up much. And since we had it under control with the SBOs now, we considered his sound sensitivity a thing of the past, but remember, we were only treating the symptoms at the time. When he was much younger, it had been debilitating enough to prevent us from visiting amusement parks or anything with constant or sporadically loud noises. I couldn't even open my car windows and listen to music louder than a talking voice, he would lose it in the back seat. It's hard to imagine this is the same child who now has to be asked to turn down the Metallica! Although these experiences were considered to be a thing of the past, they certainly weren't forgotten.

Our bodies are designed to isolate and encapsulate toxins which can be acquired externally or created endogenously (internally). Even the neurotransmitters and hormones our body creates during a stressful situation can be viewed as "toxins" by our body. The process of encapsulating toxins within the tissue structures of our body is a protective mechanism. By storing toxins, they are less available to cause further damage. When we embark on a modality that releases these stored toxins for the sake of healing, we are saturating the bloodstream once again with them in an attempt to eliminate them for good. This also means that we will see a resurgence of the symptoms associated with the release of these once stored "toxins." Once you grasp the concept of how this works within our bodies, you might be wondering how this would look in real life situations.

ONE DAY after giving Grayson one of his secretive (we weren't told what remedies we were given) homeopathic "clear" pellets, I turned our television on and the volume was accidentally left very loud. Grayson had been sitting playing beside me when a startling voice from the TV boomed through our family room, unexpectedly. He instantly cupped his ears just like old times and began wailing. After my own startled response from the unexpected surprise volume, I may have been even more astounded by Grayson's reaction.

I froze as I glanced over at him. Experiences from the past flooded my memory instantly. Fear set in.

"Grayson, did the TV scare you, I'm sorry about that buddy, I'm turning it down..." I said as I turned the volume way down.

He still wasn't removing his hands from his ears, and he was sobbing. I was surprised at his extreme reaction, which brought me right back to a day at a carnival when Grayson was five years old, and he couldn't relax or take his hands from his ears. He had climbed into his baby brother's stroller and continuously shrieked over and over that he wanted to go home, crying in panic uncontrollably. I felt my stomach sink as if I were reliving the experience. I had wanted so badly for Grayson to be able to enjoy being a child at a carnival, brightly lit games, the feeling of the wind through his hair on the rides, laughing until his stomach hurt while whirling around and around on favorite childhood rides like the Scrambler. As much pain as he was obviously experiencing, I'm sure my pain for his loss was ten times greater.

As this event unfolded in front of me in our family room, I got stuck in the past, fear took over briefly and I began to analyze the situation as I had always done in the past. Could it be candida overgrowth returning? As I would later learn, we had just given him a remedy called an "ultrasound clear." The concept of doing a homeopathic "clear" is the act of giving a remedy made from the very substance that caused a shift in health in an attempt to clear out the old energy imprint and/or toxins associated with the original exposure, which the body has actually encapsulated in an attempt to protect the host from the toxins created by, or encountered during the experience. In hindsight, I recalled discussions with others who mentioned that the ultrasound clears took care of their children's sound sensitivities and that ultrasounds are actually incredibly loud to our babies in utero, something we are never told to consider when we are so excited to "meet" our babies as they develop in their mysterious little water world.

After the aggravation that day, we never saw the sound sensitivity again, ever. We can play loud music, HE plays loud music, he loves carnivals, we can flush public toilets, he doesn't even flinch… ah the things we take for granted in life.

· · ·

SPEAKING of taking things for granted, just when things were looking so promising, after we finally found the practitioner who was able to help guide us to what felt like a higher level of healing; a surprising turn of events would rip the hope right out of my hands, and I would be left standing there empty-handed and with more difficult decisions to consider.

Little did I know that what was about to take place would also serve as the catalyst that would help facilitate a new paradigm in our healing journey, one where we began to trust and rely more on ourselves than others.

17

Lessons in disguise

TRAGIC EVENTS LEAD TO GROWTH

"Whenever something negative happens to you, there is a deep lesson concealed within."

-Eckhart Tolle

WE WERE deep into treatment with our homeopathic student, a pending appointment on the horizon, when our hopes and dreams came crashing down on us. We were left hanging for days as our appointment was first put on hold, then ultimately canceled without explanation. There were others, friends and acquaintances who were also their clients that were put on hold, although not everyone we knew was given the same message. Our treatment was being discontinued! It was utter chaos. Parents were contacting me left and right, wondering if we had been "cut" from treatment too. Some were hearing from their homeopaths that everything would be ok, to just hold tight and to be patient while they waited for "instructions." It all seemed so odd and the information was inconsistent from one homeopath to another within the same school. I wasn't hearing anything reassuring from our homeopath. I knew the instant our appointment was rescheduled, that we were just being put off.

There was a fabulous private Facebook group for all of their clients, where parents were supporting one another and sharing their unimaginable success stories. It was a place where we could get a boost of morale and share our amazing improvements or get questions answered. There was nothing like it. It shined a light of hope for parents awaiting their first appointment, and was enough to start the healing then and there. The group was instantly gone too, just like our treatment, pulled right out from under us, without explanation. Parents who were lucky enough to retain their homeopathic services were being threatened with the loss of their treatment if they contacted anyone else who had received treatment from them in the past. It was clear that they were hiding something.

Then one day, we got a generic, wordy, yet vague letter suggesting that we were involved in breaking "rules," some unwritten rules saying we couldn't talk to other homeopaths, nor could we ever consider self-treating. Most parents who seek homeopathic treatment have used remedies for acute situations or have friends who were also treating homeopathically. In fact, many of us were on Facebook groups where we discussed homeopathy regularly.

Apparently we had broken some rule or another, but our letters were all identical, so we didn't even know which rule we had supposedly broken to land us in no-treatment-land, nor were we given an opportunity to rectify whatever went wrong.

Some parents were shattered, because they were in the middle of treating serious illnesses such as seizures, and infections like MRSA. They were dumped without so much as a list of remedies their child had been on so that they could continue treatment, they couldn't even pass their treatment history on to another practitioner for continuity in treatment. It meant they would have to start over with someone new, but who could pick up where they left off without a treatment history? And how would they pick up the pieces that were left behind by this group? The damage this alone caused to some families was added to their list of stressors at an already challenging time in their lives. It was a very dark time for many parents who felt this was their chance at recovery. The long-awaited light at the end of the tunnel was suddenly gone.

WHEN I RECEIVED our letter of discontinued services, I had been waiting to reschedule my cancelled appointment. I stared at it in denial for a few long, slow minutes. Time stood still in that moment as I held my breath. I couldn't fathom how anyone could do this to a family, let alone dozens of them. It was so unprofessional and just plain hurtful. Where were their values? These were supposed to be healers, yet their behavior was contradictory to their role. What had everyone done that was so incredulous that it warranted leaving them stranded right smack in the middle of their treatment? The atrocities continued with the group, as their remaining clients clung to them, bound by strict rules that governed their actions even outside of their homeopathic treatment. As painful as it was to be left without a homeopath, I knew it was time to move on, regardless. I couldn't be reined in like a wild animal, I wouldn't. I have always followed my gut and I wouldn't stop now. If that was so wrong, then they weren't the right practitioners for me and my family. Anytime I tried to put our healing 100% in the hands of another practitioner, the Universe chewed me up and spit me out! What I didn't recognize at the time was a Divine intervention, putting me at the helm. I picked myself up, dusted myself off and kept going, like I always had.

Meanwhile, I had begun to read Bruce Lipton's "The Biology of Belief" which illuminated a great big lightbulb for me. In this book, nationally recognized cellular biologist Dr. Bruce Lipton shares his research as it relates to the structure and function of cells, but this is no boring medical book, instead he highlights the results of his research which calls into question everything we know about how our cells function. He discovers and illustrates the findings that our cells actually respond to our thoughts, quite literally! Our thoughts, which are based on our deeply rooted beliefs, are the driving force behind illness and disease. I already understood how homeopathy works and why it works, but to hear how we can potentially *become* homeopathy itself, from a Nationally known cellular biologist, was the icing on the cake. My comprehension of where we needed to be, shifted with the details in this book. It fused my perception with my goals, forging a path right in front of me.

I would again be reminded of this moment when over a year later, I was in my Reiki Master class and the instructor said, *"You ARE Reiki, you ARE energy, you ARE the crystal and it oozes from every pore of your body."*

It was time to BE healthy, to think healthy thoughts and to put the past behind us, where it belongs. Gandhi had the right idea all along, *"Be the change you want to see in the world..."* Our visions create our reality. How many times had I read this, but didn't really understand how profoundly real it was.

This had me thinking about the diagnoses we seek for our children in the name of guidance. They are necessary for insurance payments and to give us some relief from the fears we create surrounding the circumstances of our situation. But the danger in a label is that they hold us in a negative vibrational pattern. We had spent years focused on healing our boys, attempting to "fix" what was perceived as broken. Not once did we stop and think about what that must have felt like for them. The energy we poured into singling out our children as broken, and trying to repair them, was spent spinning in circles. It only served to drive us further into our pain and suffering. It was time to get off this awful ride.

I began hearing stories about children who were previously doing so well with the homeopathic college suddenly plummeting. Why? Why now? It wasn't a coincidence. What was different? Then something hit me! It dawned on me that the reason everyone was experiencing such fabulous results with the student homeopaths was because of the Facebook group support! When a group of us were dropped from treatment, they also withdrew the Facebook group. Not that the homeopathy wasn't a healing force in itself, the right remedy could certainly be miraculous, but compiled with the incredible collective consciousness that we were pouring into our days, healing was lifted up to the next level…the spiritual level.

I felt like a butterfly spreading her wings after being held tightly in a restrictive cocoon, and I knew our healing could take on this euphoric state. Suddenly I was filled with the distinct feeling that healing happens within us. I believed it, I lived it, and I finally knew this was it!! It was time to discard the victim hat.

OUR JOURNEY really started to take shape now.

18

Enlightenment

LEAVING THE LABELS BEHIND

"The next logical step, to the degree you will allow it."

-Abraham-Hicks

MY EXTENSIVE LEARNING began to take on the form of more energy work. I was drawn to reading about the chakras, the aura layers and how they affect our health. It was an enlightening period for me. Through experiences like seeing a Shaman, regular meditation and yoga, my purpose was beginning to unfold and take shape. I could actually feel the shift in my vibration to one which was much higher than even just weeks prior.

I began to look forward to my quiet meditations outside. Sitting in the sun on our back deck, I stared off at the beautiful field behind our house. The sprawling farm enveloped by hills in the distance could be so mesmerizing. My gaze drifted up to the clouds floating overhead in the wide, blue canvas sky. Many minutes ticked by as I pondered life. There was so much more out there. I felt it, I'd always felt it. What we see from this human world doesn't even scratch the surface.

From there, I went into meditation blending the healing energies from the earth and sky together within me. The warm rays of the sun felt exhilarating on my face. It fueled me further. When in this place, I felt truly invincible.

It was from moments like these that I developed and accumulated strength to trust myself. More self-awareness led me to realize that all along, I had actually been following my intuition. I was already pulling in vibrations and experiences to heal us, although threads of contradiction were woven throughout, in the form of negative thought patterns. The path before me now illuminated my newest goals.

SINCE WE HAD no practitioner at this point, I chose to just see where this could take us, rather than jumping on the bandwagon of blindly choosing another homeopath. Perhaps the path was going to present itself to me as I meandered along its unfamiliar terrain. I needed time to sort through my purpose, which felt very much like it was up to me to heal us and that it must start with me! I now knew that by healing myself at the core, my children, who are enveloped in my energy all day, would surely heal with me. We are, after all, intimately connected.

My expanding knowledge led me to muscle testing, which is a form of dowsing. I was very interested in buying a radionic machine and I was aware that one must either use a stick plate (sensing the energy flow through the fingers) or a pendulum, in order to fully take advantage of the benefits that a radionic machine had to offer. So, as I was researching the right machine for us, I practiced working with a pendulum. It was fascinating to me how I could tap into my higher self and find answers to just about anything. I began dowsing our lists of remedies and finding remedy/potency matches for us and was astounded at the progress we began to see. In fact, Grayson's tics were even diminishing in frequency and intensity, something we hadn't experienced up to this point.

Worries about the kids melted away, and I spent more time focused on the things that felt right. Even my style of home schooling began to shift. I was less worried about the technicalities of every little thing and more focused on the spirit we put into the things that made us who we were. The kids were flourishing like never before. There was just no comparison to the progress we had seen in the past. We were leaving every label and diagnosis in our rear view mirrors in an insanely fast amount of time. Thinking back to when I was in the trenches and feeling sad for myself, I noticed how the kids' behavior would follow suit, and when I was feeling hopeful again, they would trail along for that ride too. All it took was my own awareness of our intrinsic power to heal. It truly is within us!

I THOUGHT life would slow to a more peaceful pace, which it really did, for the kids anyway...but my own awakening was sailing and the spiritual downloads I was receiving would have me feeling like I was speeding down the highway of life without a seatbelt.

19

Soul searching

EXPANDING THE HEALING TOOLBOX

"When you change the way you look at things, the things you look at change."

-Wayne Dyer

WHEN I LOOK BACK on the course of events that shaped the past five years, it was glaringly obvious that our patterns and energy waxed and waned with each new reason for hope. There was no direct road to recovery. The idea of a change in treatment would always elicit great and encouraging responses, instilling a feeling of progress, only to eventually see that progress fades with time. It was becoming clear that our faith was driving the bus, not the other way around.

I extracted something from every experience, and I noticed a history of jumping from one practitioner to another. One NAET appointment here, one cranial sacral appointment there, two soul retrievals and then never again. It dawned on me that I wasn't searching for a practitioner to heal us, because every single one of these experiences did elicit a response, so if I was looking for healing direction from another person, I would have stuck it out with any one or more of these professionals. I was extracting something vital from each of these experiences and it added to the accumulative effect that would eventually smack me upside the head, when I eventually had an appointment for myself with our energy healer, and she told me that my purpose was to heal Grayson. ME! Not a doctor, healer or practitioner, but me, his mother.

It all suddenly made sense. It wasn't that I hadn't connected with anything we tried, instead it was quite the opposite, I was connecting with all of our experiences. It was essential to building up my foundation. Even a well-built house needs a strong, stable foundation. I was drawn to each experience with purpose. The modalities and practitioners weren't intended to become our crutch, they were the result of my intuitive navigation system functioning on autopilot.

You might be thinking, "Well, how are you going to do it all, how can you become the equivalent of all those modalities and practitioners?" The thing was, I didn't need to duplicate their efforts. What they all brought to my healing tool box (and reiterated for me) was a common denominator of belief. My children were responders to just about every modality we tried, because I chose to believe in them. Just like the homeopathic student treatment, the healing modality alone wasn't where the progress was coming from, my power in the situation was how strongly I believed in it. Suddenly, Bruce Lipton's book was describing my own life, and it was all coming together. My belief system was shifting from physical to spiritual, it was moving from the surface of my conscious mind to the subconscious now. THIS is where the healing is.

When you feel something so pure and real in your soul, you KNOW there is nothing else possible. This knowing comes from within. I had spent years cultivating this inner strength, but now it would have the opportunity to shine.

THE REAL BONUS became clear that in addition to healing my children, I was suddenly profoundly aware of my own needs and desires, as well as my own health requirements. I wasn't just healing them, I was healing myself and vice versa. Every family member was intimately tied to one another, every behavior, every craving, and every experience shaped the entire family unit. We all moved fluidly together, or sometimes not so fluidly, but always shifting together in and out of our emotions and actions like waves lapping on the sand. It was time for me to focus on me, it was my turn to be on the front burner. And as a result, I could expect to also see improvement in the rest of my household.

My first goal was to fulfill a lofty dream I had. I wanted a radionic machine. I knew it would be something that would take time for me to master and might even require a learning curve that could require the rest of my life to truly become proficient at. The potential uses for a radionic machine spans the globe, quite literally! I could even send healing to someone halfway around the world, if I wanted. I know, I know…if you are catching on to my learning curve already, you are right to think that I AM the radionic machine. The way I think of a machine like this is not one which replaces my intuition, but rather a method of enhancing my intuition and capabilities. It becomes an extension of myself. In my own personal opinion, without intent, the radionic machine is useless. With a database of over 20,000 frequencies available for the purpose of making or sending frequency/homeopathic treatments, it expanded my vision beyond my knowledge. Now, it was time to catch up with that vision.

I had a driving desire to learn, fast and furiously. I often had five books open at one time, plus a class of some sort going on. As I was taking these various classes to learn more and reading umpteen books, I was using the learned techniques that resonated with me, to balance our life as a whole.

ONE OF THE more useful self-help energy healing techniques I learned was Reiki. I know it's pretty common for Reiki to be the first step to a successful awakening and I can see why now. I tend to be pretty resistant to anything "everyone else" is doing, but I decided it was time to be open to whatever came across my path. I was already using hands-on techniques I learned in Reconnective Healing, but Reiki was a nice addition and the attunements (which are like spiritual initiations) that are part of each level of Reiki, always seemed to be just enough to push me over the edge, a push that I needed each time. It's amazing how timing always worked out for me when I allowed the flow of life to gently nudge me without trying to force or resist it. A lot transpired for me in the period between being certified in Reiki level one, level two, and Reiki Master.

REIKI IS A FORM OF NON-INVASIVE, hands-on energy work that has an impact on the human subtle energy system, by harmonizing energies that may be otherwise incompatible. If your "life force energy" is low, you will be more susceptible to illness and stress. Reiki strengthens this life force, restoring the patient's physical and emotional well-being. Each method carries a unique vibrational frequency and will create different effects. It is encouraging to learn that Reiki has been used in at least seventy six hospitals, medical clinics and hospice programs as a standard part of care!

JENNA GALLIGANI, who is a psychotherapist and Reiki Master (and also happens to be my sister-in-law) explains it well for her Reiki students. Below is an excerpt from her student's literature.

What is Reiki?

Reiki is translated as "universal energy." Reiki uses the transfer of energy through a "laying of the hands" on the individual in a variety of hand positions that promote relaxation, reduction of physical symptoms/illnesses, and improved emotional health. The energy transfer is believed to come from the life force that flows within each of us. This life force has many names in different cultures such as Chi in China, Prana in India, or Ki in Japan.

The life force flows through all living beings, plants, and objects such as rocks or crystals. The life force illuminates our organs and brings health and optimal function to them.

When our life force is low then this causes our organs and systems to function at a lower level thus creating illness and disease. To recharge our life force we need proper sleep, food, sun, grounding from the earth, and our breath. The life force leaves the body when one dies. The higher our life force, then the better we feel and the better we function.

Reiki assists us in channeling this life force by drawing it from our environment so that we do not drain our own. As one becomes a conductor between the environment/universe, we allow the flow of this energy to transmit through us and to others. Reiki energy helps to then raise the life force, which in turns aids in the body's natural ability to heal.

Quantum Physics says that everything is energy whether a living being, plant, or object. The smallest part of matter is an atom. Within an atom there are vortexes of energy that are in constant motion. This energy within the atom has also been demonstrated to be able to communicate to other atoms without physically touching the other atom to exchange the information. Quantum Physics has shown again and again the evidence that this energy exists within all atoms therefore declaring that all things are made of energy.

The energy within the atoms vibrate at different rates creating a certain input to our senses. A physical hard surface has a different vibrational pattern than a liquid and both have a different vibration than a gas. These different vibrational patterns provide physical properties such as a hard surface of a table, cold water, a soft blanket, etc. Our senses then interpret the vibration so that we experience the table as a table, the water as water,

and the blanket as a blanket. Our senses interpret these vibrations, which provides us with information such as what something looks like, what it feels like, what it sounds like, etc.

There are many energies that are not able to be seen or heard by the human eye or ear, yet we know the energy exists due to the impact of this energy. Now, we have many types of machines and devices that help us to detect various types of energy such as SQUID magnetometer (reads the bio magnetic field around the body), EKG (records the electrical signals of the heart), EEG (records the electrical signals of the brain), and ultrasound (uses sound waves to create an image, etc.).

In summary, everything is energy. Different energies carry different vibrational patterns. Certain vibrational patterns can influence each other such as a glass of lemonade with ice. The two variations in temperature will eventually combine into a temperature somewhere between the two opposing temperatures. The theory with Reiki is that the universal energy has a higher vibration so that as a practitioner transfers this energy into the client it raises the vibration of the client thus it stimulates the life force energy to engage the body's natural healing process.

Examples of energy that is unseen, yet we feel the effect In nature:

- *Gravity Air*
- *Trees giving off oxygen*
- *The earth's electromagnetic field Sound from thunder traveling*
- *Light from lightning traveling faster than the thunder Carbon monoxide from a fire*

Manmade devices:

- *Radio frequencies Cell phones*
- *The Electro Magnetic Fields that appliances and cell phones give off Wi-fi*
- *The vibration felt when an instrument is played Microwave ovens*

As YOU CAN SEE, we encounter energetic frequencies daily without conscious awareness. Science has successfully harnessed this energy for diagnostic and technological purposes such as ultrasound technology and laser surgery. The conscious realization that this energy existed and could be used to our benefit was very powerful, and with time, my own purpose and awareness began to shift with this acknowledgement.

The power of manifestation

YOU ARE WHAT YOU BELIEVE

"*What you think, you become. What you feel, you attract. What you imagine, you create.*"

-Buddha

GOING BACK to the idea that a label carries its own frequency, when we identify with a label or a diagnosis, and don't release possible fears and emotions tied to that label, we are constantly saturated by the frequencies of this dis-ease daily. Think about the impact this has on us and our children. Have you ever noticed that most of the cancer patients who die, sadly do so following a diagnosis? It's rare that a person dies and then it's discovered that they died from cancer. In fact, many people die with cancer in their bodies, although not from the cancer itself. So why does the health of many cancer patients decline immediately following their diagnosis?

There is a phenomenon known as negative manifestation. Now, I know you are thinking, there is no way that a cancer patient is only dying because of his or her diagnosis. Well, that is a discussion for another book, quite frankly, because cancer patients generally have one thing in common emotionally, which is suppressed negative emotions and/or toxins that were never dealt with. For the sake of staying on topic, a negative manifestation is the burden of a negative thought, basically akin to being told over and over again that you will amount to nothing. This is a well-known phenomenon even in psychology, studied and proven time and again. If you fall prey to this manifestation, and you allow yourself to believe it by developing fears and expectations associated with it, you might live this "truth" and actually end up amounting to nothing, because you believe it! Accumulate enough of these negative manifestation/frequencies and you will be surrounded by them, weighing you down, pulling you down.

Let's envision a child with the diagnosis of PANDAS. What instantly comes to mind when you think of this dis-ease, even if you have never personally experienced it for yourself? A child with an autoimmune disease and its associated with a pathogen commonly referred to as strep, right? So, picture in your mind, if you will, a child who receives this diagnosis and his parents now identify their child with this disorder, very much like the unfortunate child who is led to believe he will amount to nothing. Can you see the manifestations/frequencies surrounding the child's and parent's aura? Clear as day, I see "strep" in the aura, and I see the body attacking itself. And whether it was truly there or not from the beginning, it sure is there now.

If we go back to the Law of Attraction, a simple concept that we attract like-frequencies, as in the child who grows up amounting to nothing, because he believes what he is told repeatedly by his parents, what is going to happen to the PANDAS child? How is this child going to release these negative manifestations and overcome them, if his own parents can't? It's a vicious cycle and who do you think has to stop this pattern from repeating? That's right, it must start with the parents!!

Now be careful here, because this is NOT blame, this is meant to highlight awareness. We can only change that which we are aware of. No one should ever blame themselves for not knowing something earlier. Blame is a very low vibration emotion and it just serves to depress the system with negative manifestations, yet again. So, let's move on up to a higher frequency emotion and get out of this trap! How can you do that, you ask? There are numerous ways to increase your vibration, as well as your child's.

Often, when you increase your own vibration, your child who is engulfed in your frequencies by sheer exposure, will begin to shift with you, but if you need help, there are many well-known methods of raising your vibration that can be shared with your child either directly or by exposure to your shift. For example, homeopathy, which crosses over into energy medicine, yup that's right, it balances your vibration by exposing you to beneficial frequencies and/or neutralizing damaging frequencies! Meditation is a personal favorite of mine, and children can benefit greatly from understanding how meditation can help them. For children, start with mindfulness practices, then move up to meditation in short spurts, as they can tolerate sitting still. I have always loved guided meditation for kids, it is easier for them to close their eyes and focus on a soft voice, than to sit suspended in silence for periods of time. Reiki is a great neutral form of raising your vibration. You can either go to a practitioner, or even better, why pay someone else to do what you can do quite easily yourself? Classes are widely available and it's not a time consuming practice to learn. Crystals share their heightened frequencies with you when exposed to them regularly. You can even find crystals specific to your needs. Structured water carries higher, healthy vibrations and surrounds and penetrates your cells with these hydrating energetic atoms. QiGong, yoga and martial arts, the list is endless. In the case of a child like the PANDAS child referred to above, simply and consciously highlighting their positive attributes will raise the vibration around both of you. Your reality is created by your focus and intention. Find something that resonates with you, pun intended, (wink) and expand on it, working it into your lifestyle routines.

I'D LIKE to share an experience that really solidified this

phenomenon for me. I was already quite aware of the quantum physics behind the idea of the Law of Attraction, but to see it play out in this way was eye-opening and incredibly confirming. Our younger son, Gavin, is quite an empath, he is even telepathic and we are often surprised by the experiences we share with him, resulting from his amazing unadulterated awareness of the energy around him. As I was writing this book, an Ebola scare had the nation in a tizzy about exposure to its venomous grip and its resulting death. The tension on social media was quite evident with postings by the droves with the latest buzz words about who the next unlucky victims were and, of course, this equated to a lot of frightened people, because it left them feeling exposed and helpless. They feared they could easily be the next victims if they so much as looked at an Ebola victim accidentally.

It was quite unsettling, even for a person like me who believes we have the power to heal from anything, if it's not our time to go. I allowed myself to get caught up in the media hype at times, fearing for the poor victims who didn't have a chance at recovering from such a deadly pathogen and wondered how easily it might be able to reach out and touch us too. I began to document holistic and home-opathic ways to combat Ebola should we ever encounter someone with it, "just in case." Around this time, Gavin had been behaving like he was coming down with something, he was sluggish and moody, his nose was stuffy off and on, so I ran a quick diagnostic on my radionic machine to see what viruses might be implicated and you would not believe the virus that came in at the top of the list. Ebola! Clearly he did NOT contract actual Ebola while we were home schooling in our little bubble world. We had not traveled anywhere to suggest he could actually contract the virus on a phys-ical level. He certainly wasn't exhibiting any of the real symptoms. Yet, ironically, when I gave him a single homeopathic dose of the matching frequencies to this virus, he got a bloody nose and his health moved towards vibrant health again.

Ebola is typified by the unique symptom of hemorrhaging from the orifices. So, what would cause this possible frequency connection in his body? Law of Attraction, of course!! Was it just me bringing those frequencies into his environment or could it be a situation where collective consciousness was drawing it in on a larger scale? Perhaps I was his conduit from the collective consciousness to his own immediate surroundings.

If we expand on this concept of large scale manifestation, the idea of collective or global consciousness is that we generate more power in our intent if it's multiplied by the number of people in that vibration, at the same time. The Global Consciousness Project is a large scale project that has been tracking data for over a decade. During the World Trade Center attacks, they were able to compile data suggesting that in our collective consciousness, we were already aware of the attack 4-5 hours before it occurred. They experienced significant peaks and valleys through the course of this horrific event. The effects can clearly go both directions. We can piggyback off of the elevating frequencies of beneficial thoughts or vibrations, like when a group of people meditate together, especially when they meditate on a common theme. But what if a group of people get caught up in a negative pattern of thought? Think about the consequences…and I believe this is happening on a smaller scale when families are surrounding their children with a label, any kind of negative label. They are joining the collective consciousness associated with that label. And it's these very labels that are demanding change.

AUTISM AND PANDAS/PANS are the boiling point of this change. It is human nature to wait until we are heavily motivated to make change. We don't just wake up one day and say, "I think I need to do something different today…" well, most of us don't anyway. We need to be inspired to change and sometimes that inspiration must come in the way of what feels like a painful dead end. If I didn't discover that my child must eat a diet free of gluten, dairy and soy to feel well, do you think I would have removed them (and 20 other foods) from his diet overnight, complicating our lives for no reason? Heck no! Would I choose to wake up every three hours all night, on the weekends just for fun, or did I need to be inspired to try oral chelation for overt heavy metal toxicities? But on the other side of this coin, would I be living a much healthier and enriched life today without our child to inspire me? I wouldn't wish Autism or PANDAS/PANS on anyone, but I can say without a doubt, that I am grateful for the turn of events due to these experiences in our lives.

With the sheer size of the Autism and PANDAS/PANS communities, think of the power we can elicit, if we spin this epidemic to benefit us. The power of the masses can change the world as we see it today. This is what awareness is all about. And frankly, I am beginning to believe that this is the purpose of Autism and PANDAS/PANS. We have been given the opportunity to use the lessons we've learned through our experiences to make a difference.

On a smaller scale, has it become more clear to you now why families who use healing modalities like homeopathy see such amazing results? The family is saturating that child, and themselves, with the belief that the child is going to heal. Many say you don't have to fully believe in homeopathy for it to work, but I beg to differ, because if a person is trying homeopathy, even reluctantly, there IS a piece of them that believes, even if it's just in the form of hope. Hope holds a higher vibration than guilt and blame. You are already moving up the scale to health by residing at this emotion rather than the blame trap emotion.

A LOT of people want to know who I recommend as an energy healing practitioner or homeopath and this is something I struggle with answering each time. When someone wants direction such as who to see and what methods to trust, I want to help, it's my nature to help…but part of me feels like this would be a form of steering the person onto a path that may not be meant for them. One could argue that if they are in contact with me to begin with, they ARE on their path, and I whole heartedly agree, but I also think that when we reach these sort of forks in the road, my role is less about steering them down one particular path and more about reminding them to open their heart to the intuition that speaks to them about these decisions.

So, if you were to ask me what I recommend, I have been known to suggest that you put your desires out into the Universe and wait to see how the path unfolds before you. You will receive signs and if you are open to them, following those signs will reveal what is meant to be, whether that is a practitioner, type of modality or a next step for you and your child(ren). This may be hard for many to grasp, because it's all right-brained. It also requires a lot of patience and trust that you will receive what you are asking for. You have to get out of your conscious, analytical mind and let go of the expectations. Create a vision (whether it be physical or mental) and trust it.

21

Transforming worrisome thoughts

"Worrying does not empty tomorrow of its troubles, it empties today of its strength."

-Corrie Ten Boom

HAVING A CHILD with what is perceived as a chronic illness also means that worrisome thought patterns are commonplace. It's easy to get caught up in the fears of what will happen to your child as s/he ages, as you age, and even more frightening, when you are gone. And I certainly don't mean to diminish these very real and for many, looming concerns. It is very important to plan, but I want to shed light on the distinction between planning (taking steps to address the concern) and spending wasted energy on worrying about it. Worry is the result of a thought projection into the future about the unknown. We use the information we have today, combined with our perception and thought patterns from our past, to devise feelings of uncertainty, anxiety and thoughts of being threatened. These thought patterns alone can release the same chemicals (adrenaline, cortisol, etc) that would be released during the actual event, as if it were really happening right now. It seems pretty obvious that by avoiding counterproductive thoughts, we can avoid the stress trigger, but how do we do that?

While reading the children's book series "Sara" by Esther and Jerry Hicks to my boys, we learned step-by-step basics about the Law of Attraction. There is no easier way to learn something than to go back to the basics and what better way than to use the same language we use to teach children?

We learned that we must define what we do NOT want, which seems simple enough, right? After all, this part comes quite natural for most of us! The key distinction is to not get stuck here though, which is where our worrisome thoughts have a chance to take root and form a life of their own. Instead, we must only use this as information, to define what we DO want. Once we have that figured out and we fully understand what we do want, it's time to immerse yourself in the feelings of that thought. Go there, FEEL it, as if it is true. Now you are vibrating as if it were true!

By continuing to bring out what you do what, you are attracting the positive vibration into your reality and you will continue to attract this vibration into your life. Quite simply, your gauge becomes how you feel. By focusing on what you want, your continuing efforts will also be directed at what you want. If your focus is on what you don't want, or the gap between what you do and don't want, your frequency will reflect those thoughts and feelings. Remember, your body doesn't know the difference between what is real and what is perceived.

It does take some effort to master, but with time and practice, old thought patterns can be changed.

I'VE ALWAYS CONSIDERED myself to be fairly effective at living in the here and now, that is, until I gave birth to children who challenged everything I thought I knew about myself. And isn't that also the beauty of having children? They change us profoundly, hopefully for the better. We become more in touch with ourselves while learning who they are. The growing pains of this process can be overwhelming at times, but if you just continue to focus on what you want, the outcome is bound to be more positive than the alternative.

The idea that we attract what we put out can easily be explained by the old saying, "Birds of a feather flock together." Think about the company you keep. How is it related to what you attract? When I began seeking answers for our recovery, I found myself attracting the very people who would teach me what I needed to know in order to see the recovery I envisioned. My circle of friends slowly moved towards those I could relate to and even more importantly, those I could learn from. The more I put my desires out there, the more I kept that feeling of what I was aiming for, the more I attracted exactly what I needed to reach my goal.

THE POWER of social media puts these connections right at our fingertips. By surrounding myself with like-minded people, my own strength improved. The more my strength improved, the more the kids improved. I can't stress this enough, it is very important to reduce negativity and increase positivity. This must include the company you keep.

Thankfully, this will almost inevitably work itself out based on the Law of Attraction, but you must be prepared to go with the flow in order to see the results. By changing yourself, your surroundings will naturally change. Resistance will block improvement, whereas joining the flow of whatever is brought your way can result in miraculous shifts.

MY FIRST PROFOUND and obvious experience with this theory was when we were struggling with Grayson's continual facial tics. Nothing had worked to resolve them entirely and seeing them regularly was a constant reminder of what we didn't want. It was so easy to just keep thinking about what we didn't want, heck, it was right there in our faces (written all over his face), reminding us daily! Somewhere along the way, I made the decision to stop giving energy to the negative feeling his tics elicited in me. I decided to focus on him being tic-free, PANDAS/PANS-free. I didn't just believe this for myself, I actually began telling people that it was all behind us, that we were no longer dealing with PANDAS/PANS. It felt as if I was also telling Grayson's body that he didn't resonate with it any longer.

One day, I noticed that his tics were gone! His tics had previously changed form and even reduced significantly at times, but they never went away entirely like this! Tics tend to be his first sign that something is up, whether it is a pending illness, stress, mold exposure, or pollen triggers, so although they do occasionally return, I know without a shadow of a doubt, that they will also rescind. I no longer give energy to them.

Sometimes a solution or an intervention is necessary, like a homeopathic remedy, but the difference is in the energy that surrounds the decision. I don't choose a remedy from a place of panic. I choose one from a place of centered understanding of the situation. The tics are gone more than they are active, and even when they are active, they are mild enough that the average person wouldn't even pick up on them. They generally communicate to us that he is coping with a stressor of some sort and it allows us to be aware, but not concerned. Instead, I am now thankful that I have a way to gauge when he is struggling with something.

It was important to make some major changes in my life in order to see this through. One of those changes was to move away from the claws of diagnosis that were trying to hold us back. I had been so deeply immersed in many Autism and PANDAS/PANS Facebook groups that I was regularly swimming in the energy of the diagnosis. Belonging to this community of fellow Autism and PANDAS/PANS parents served an important purpose in our lives, but their time had an expiration. I needed to break free from the prison of labels and move toward our goal, toward what we wanted to attract. I decided to step down as moderator in a group I had created on Facebook so that I could stay focused on attracting more of what we needed to fulfill recovery. It was a hard decision to make, because I felt a responsibility to the members. Instead of feeling like I was giving up on them, I chose to communicate our journey from the angle that perhaps I would give people hope, something to aim for themselves. This is what I wrote to the group as I bowed out gracefully to move onto the next chapter of healing:

I would like to make an announcement.

I announce this with conflicting sadness and joy, but I will be leaving It Takes a Fanatic (and all Autism and PANDAS groups for that matter). This is a choice I didn't make lightly.

Let me explain where I am. My family and I have left Autism and PANDAS in our dust. My family is on the fast track to recovery and my belief system which has done a 360, was the foundation for clearing the last hurdle. I am in a place where moving on with the rest of our lives is our next step. In order to move forward, I must eliminate the daily energy of "Autism" and "PANDAS" from our lives.

I don't want anyone here to think I am giving up on you, quite the contrary, I am still here, still on FB and still believe in helping. I do this with a different approach now though. I know that people who are drawn to me will find me, it's the Law of Attraction at work.

I am relieved to be freed from the confines of Autism and PANDAS, so I am going to break free entirely, for me and for my family. I am not disconnecting from my Autism friends, I am so grateful for each and every one of you, I am just eliminating the daily communication which brings me back to the Autism/PANDAS energy.

I am writing a book and hope to get through that before moving on to my next "project", hahaha. Only time will tell where my energy is going to be best used. I have many dreams and I plan to begin fulfilling them now.

Remember, Autism and PANDAS are reversible!! Just know this in your heart and soul, regardless of what protocols you choose to try. Don't get caught up in the fear, always see this as a winning battle and you will cross the finish line. Remain in faith and hope, I wish you all the best. Stay in touch!!

––––––––––

EMBARKING on a more conscious manifestation using the Law of Attraction was not only beneficial for our children, it was also a useful tool to have in my own toolbox. To walk the talk meant that I must attempt to apply what I was learning to my own life as well. I must apply my understanding even to areas of my life that didn't involve healing my children. It was time for me to heal more fully.

THERE WAS a time when I felt like an outsider in my own neighborhood. We live at the end of a cul-de-sac where there are over a dozen children who are friends with our boys. The street we live on is a very tight-knit community of families. The parents all sat around together in the street on nice days while the children played around them. I would sit inside watching them talking and laughing while playing it out in my mind that they wouldn't like me, because we were so different from the average family. History said so, but meanwhile, I wanted nothing more than to be a part of the obvious friendships they had developed. The isolation of Autism combined with my past experiences (I felt very different growing up as the poor kid in a wealthy town, while living with my grandparents) prevented me from including myself in their established circle. We were the new kids on the block, but had lived there for years during the worst of Grayson's health so we had become very isolated and as time passed, it felt less likely that I could leap into the crowd.

"Bye Mom!" The storm door slammed behind Grayson as he ran out the front door to play with his friends. Bittersweet feelings coursed through my veins as I watched him run to meet his friends outside. On one hand, I was so very proud of his progress, he had come so far. He was socializing more appropriately and he was accepted by the children in our neighborhood, what more could I ask for? Then, why was I still feeling displaced? My gaze shifted to the parents who were sitting together out front.

This time the back door slammed, *"Mom?"* Gavin ran in, *"Can we go play basketball?"*

Of course, I wanted to say yes, because I wanted nothing more than to let them play down the street with their friends, but hesitation crept into my mind. Playing basketball down the street meant I couldn't see them from where I was sitting. It meant I would have to sit outside. My gaze shifted again to the neighbors enjoying each other's company and then back to my pending coursework on my lap. I had made a habit of completing my school work while the boys were playing within view out front. It was the perfect time to focus on school, while they were busy.

"Mom?!" Gavin broke through my thoughts again with impatience, *"Can I go play basketball with the other kids? EVERYONE else is going?"*

If I said no, I would be isolating them. I slowly nodded yes, which felt abrasive to my spirit, but then proceeded to transplant myself and my school work to the front yard within sight of the boys. Off they went, right where they belonged, with other kids, out in the gorgeous sun. There it was again, that conflicted feeling. I was so happy for them, our neighborhood had been a true blessing for them. Being homeschooled meant socializing required more effort. Living here has given them something I could never have given them myself, life experiences and friends outside of our family bubble. I am so grateful for this.

I glanced up from my schoolwork to see a few of the parents laughing. Their connection was so obvious. Why couldn't I bring myself to join them?

I was instantly brought back to memories from middle school. We had just moved in with my grandparents while my mother "sorted things out." What was initially expected to be a temporary situation became more than ten years of cramming the four of us into my grandmother's humble home in an affluent town in Connecticut. It was my first week in yet another new school. I didn't know how long we would be here, since there was nothing certain about our situation. This wasn't our first move either. I struggled with our last move too. The kids in that neighborhood were outwardly mean to me for being the new kid on the block. They even chased me through the streets on their bikes, chastising me verbally, trying to scare me...which they often succeeded at doing, but I wouldn't let it show. This move was different though, I was a little older and the kids weren't outwardly mean per say, but their avoidance of me spoke volumes.

Names were being called as each team chose their next team-mate for dodgeball. I looked at my feet while I nervously played with my fingernails. *"Jeremy!"* screamed the team captain and the whole team hooted and hollered over their newly acquired prize team-mate. *"Suzie!"* the other team captain retorted confidently, and Suzie strutted across the floor making faces at the other team who whooped at her. I began to sweat. I hated attention and the worst thing that could happen to me would be to be the last one standing in the middle of the gymnasium, because no one wanted me on their team. I didn't have the insight yet to see this from their perspective, that I was a new kid in class, injected into their lives halfway through the year after they had already made their friends. Sure enough, every other student was chosen and I was the result of the process of elimination so I quietly walked to my team, the team that didn't want me was now my team. I tried to tell myself it didn't matter and I walked with my head up. It stung but it wasn't the last of my experiences of feeling left out. This pattern repeated many times throughout my life. I was attracting what I was putting out into the Universe.

Audible laughter broke through my train of thought, which tugged me back to my front yard, where I was sitting with my school work on my lap, my shield. I could hide behind my work with dual-ity. It needed to get done, but it also protected me from feeling completely vulnerable too. So I dove in and began working.

It wasn't until one day when one of my neighbors actually asked me why I didn't like them. Why I didn't like THEM? Her words played through my mind over and over until it hit me like a ton of bricks, I had created my own situation and I was sitting smack dab in the middle of my mind-identified, low vibration situation. I had decided I was unwelcome, not the other way around. I had assumed that because we are different, we lived so very differently from anyone on this street, that we wouldn't be accepted, so of course the vibration was perpetuated by my own state of mind. I had actually manifested exactly what I was putting my attention on. I felt differ-ent, therefore, I was. My body didn't know the difference between what was real and my own thoughts. Eckhart Tolle summed it up pretty well when he wrote,

"The voice in the head has a life of its own. Most people are possessed by thought, by the mind. And since the mind is conditioned by the past, you are forced to reenact the past again and again…they are alienated from themselves as well as from others and the world around them."

I immediately decided to change my thoughts and literally overnight my situation changed too. In fact, the very next day many of my neighbors and their kids were hanging out in our front yard with us as the kids all played in a kiddie pool. Nothing like this had ever happened in all the years we lived here.

Even though we were very different from our neighbors, we have since developed mutually respectful and caring relationships. And to quote Eckhart Tolle again, the secret of happiness requires *"making peace with the present moment. The present moment is the field on which the game of life happens…"*

THERE IS nothing more true or more important.

THERE WAS a time when recovery felt eminent, now recovery was real, but it didn't come from purely focusing on the physical body, as I once thought it would. It came from tuning into the whole picture from a physical, mental and spiritual perspective. It involved the whole family and it improved the whole family. As I mentioned earlier, our state of mind emits its own vibrational pattern and the illustration below depicts this scale according to frequency. To reiterate Eckhart Tolle's comment that *"Thoughts have their own range of frequencies, with negative thoughts at the lower end of the scale and positive thoughts at the higher"* supports this illustration. To capitalize on what that looks like in everyday life, he also brilliantly said,

"All negativity is caused by an accumulation of psychological time and denial of the present. Unease, anxiety, tension, stress, worry - all forms of fear - are caused by too much future, and not enough presence. Guilt, regret, resentment, grievances, sadness, bitterness, and all forms of non-forgiveness are caused by too much past, and not enough presence."

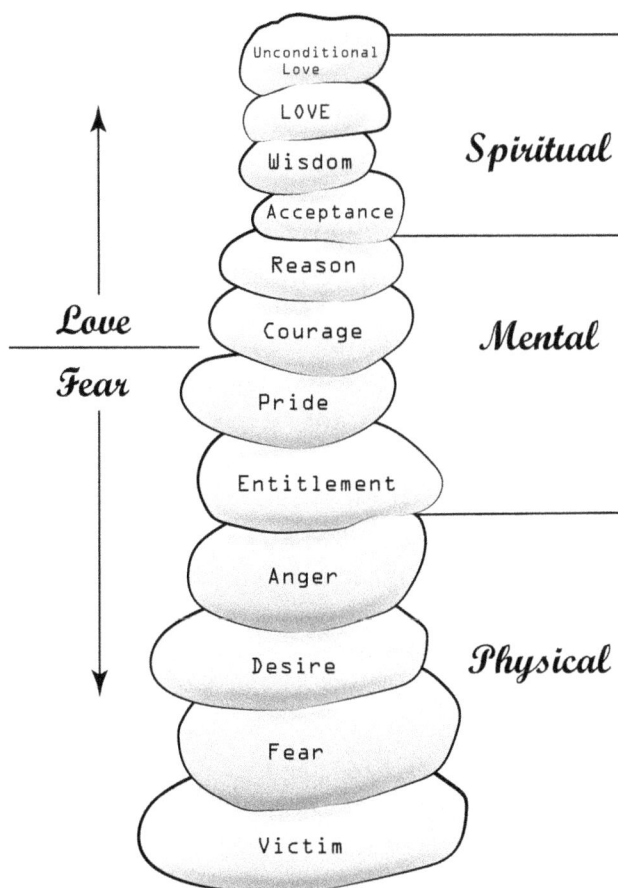

When you take some time to sit with the details and ramifications of this illustration as it relates to your own life, it can be enlightening. Cairns represent an effort to balance energies. It wasn't until I was at this point in our journey when I recognized that we had been inadvertently climbing this ladder all along. Our quest was ever-so-slowly carrying us up the rungs of consciousness, our lessons had rewritten our destiny, for me especially. I was profoundly changed by Autism and as much as I despised the pain it caused, I would rather focus on the truth, which is that Autism and PANDAS made me a better person. The story this image represented in our lives goes like this…

I BEGAN our journey as the **victim**, at the very bottom, which is also the lowest vibration. My perception was that our child and family were victims of mainstream medicine's flawed system. Vaccination harmed him and pharmaceutical approaches were all they had to offer us which left me feeling invisible and frightened.

Initially, I was paralyzed with **fear**, unsure of what to do next, practically unable to move forward. I had an intense **desire** to see my child healthy again, but how? Who could I trust? It felt like I could trust no one, and I was **angry** at the doctors who I blamed for harming him.

This anger fueled **entitlement** in me. I knew we were entitled to recovery, our child was entitled to health, and I researched and found answers, but this also encouraged **pride** to bubble up. I felt like I knew the answers, I was going to take Autism down like a warrior. This was the ugly me, the one who thought she had all the answers. Our child was getting better which inadvertently fueled this pride. With every improvement, the pride grew. I am so glad I didn't get stuck here, because I had confused pride with my ability to control his illness.

With time, I discovered that I wasn't controlling the illness, it was controlling me! Life had become all about Autism and fighting. Fighting the symptoms, fighting the pathogenic microbes, fighting the system. I didn't want to fight anymore, it felt wrong, it felt counterproductive. The machine-gun leaves carnage in its wake and when I tapped into my intuition and trusted my gut feelings, I realized we needed to work on building up and not tearing down. This is where the big changes began to take place, where the magic happened.

When I developed the **courage** to let go and trust myself more, I was able to see Autism for what it really was. It was the result of a toxic environment which took generations to develop, mentally, physically and spiritually. It took courage to sit back and wait for signs from the Universe to guide me, it took courage to trust that everything would be ok, and it took courage to believe in my intuition. It became blatantly obvious that negative emotions didn't serve us well. When I am angry, I am not the best parent I can be, I snap at people around me and when I am angry, my children are angry. How could it be that he was recovering, but we were angry all the time? It seemed like the ultimate contradiction.

With a foundation of courage, I was able to **reason** with myself and I was able to trust what would come next. It didn't look anything like the previous "me" who had forced healing at the hand of a machine-gun. I was now learning to **accept** who we were as a family and how this played into Grayson's illness and recovery. A big part of recovery was to develop acceptance, please don't mistake this for weakness, acceptance takes strength. I didn't accept and give up, I accepted and trusted, but I still acted on things that required action. With that came the **wisdom** to see more clearly. I developed a true heartfelt compassion fueled by **love** for all of human kind, even for the misinformed doctors out there. My perspective shifted and I began to see the world so very differently.

I now know that we are all right where we are meant to be, no matter how painful or difficult. We are always on a path of learning and we have the power to live the lives we want to live. I have my child's Autism to thank for my true comprehension of **unconditional love**, which I enjoy spreading far and wide. My children have also grown enormously through our experiences and will be more emotionally prepared for the world when they are ready to journey into creating their own storybooks. So where do we go from here?

22

Letting go

THE TRANSITION INTO ADOLESCENCE

"*Happiness is not something ready made, it comes from your own actions.*"

-Dalai Lama

NATURALLY, as our boys age, they explore their boundaries (and ours) more and more. This is a coming of age rite of passage for all children as they work to claim their own age- appropriate independence. We often anticipate this phase to be full of lessons for our children about the hard knocks of life and about priorities, as they begin to find their place in the world.

As their mother, I found myself inadvertently wanting to hold on tighter to my boys, because they were consciously letting go of our hands more often while they tested their wings. I have always fiercely protected them and now it was time for me to find my own strength in letting go. As our boys began to see their place in the world, their own story started to take shape. This was the time for a transition where we would give and take, push and pull and new balance was ultimately established. They want more control over their lives as they form their own visions for themselves. My world had been about holding the reigns to their health for so long, and it provided us the stability of consistency and predictability, but I must grow with them, if I truly wanted to help and support them.

The time to experiment with letting go of the reigns is while they are still comfortably surrounded by the safety of our nest. While it may appear like they are going backwards during times of exploration, this is an important experience and we must resist the desire to grab hold of their lives every step of the way. They must develop their own sense of trust through the learning curve. If you think back to the very beginning of your own journey, you will likely remember the hills and valleys of your path. They were not without purpose!

Sometimes mini experiments will take place without your awareness and hindsight will shed light on the lessons at hand. We had one such experience with Grayson at twelve. At first, I felt wildly out of control and it had me grasping at anything to gain that control again. It triggered some fears which made way for a few unsightly emotions. This is precisely where Grayson's and my lessons intersected once again, making way for a new, more enlightened, path forward.

"IT'S GAGGING ME, Mom.!! I CAN'T eat it, it's GROOOOSS!" Grayson sharply blurted from his seat at the kitchen table as he literally spit out a bite of his grass-fed, organic burger onto his plate. He has always loved burgers, I couldn't make sense of what was going on. I had wracked my brain trying to understand why his burger was so "gross" when he had eaten a burger at a restaurant just the night before, and he did so with joy, I might add!

Was it the salt? No, he loved salt and frequently reapplied more to his own dish. Nothing else was different. This problem had been progressing for the past few weeks. One by one, he was rejecting his usual favorites, but oddly, he also wasn't interested in anything new that I tried tirelessly to create from their restricted ingredient list.

Old habits die hard, so it's not surprising to me now that my old patterns surfaced temporarily, and my thoughts spiraled into the projected future…"What next? What would I do if he couldn't even have the only foods I could feed him?" I began to fear that new sensitivities were developing. In hindsight, I could see how I was stuck in the future, creating a situation that had not even played out yet. Luckily, a book I had been reading at the time "The Power of Now" by Echart Tolle, was fresh in my mind and influenced me to consciously work at staying present. Then it hit me! I replayed the very situation that held the key to the solution. He had no problem eating a burger out at a restaurant but wouldn't eat the same kind of burger at home. This felt vaguely familiar and reminded me of the days when he was self- limiting to gluten and dairy. It's the food!! While eating out, he was experiencing cross- contamination from the food in the restaurants.

Over the previous six months, we began to follow his lead and were letting him eat out more often, at his request. He became forceful in his desire to eat out with us. We resisted for a long time, resulting in outright resentment, so we decided to give in occasionally, and those occasional moments became much more frequent, as we assumed that he was handling it well. What started out as (what we thought) a harmless bite here or there turned into full meals. We even noticed a giddy-like high that came with his realization that he would get to enjoy a meal out with us. This would prove to be one of the things that led me down the path of discovering what was actually going on. This may appear like a failure on our part, but as you will soon see, it was actually an imperative lesson in disguise for all of us, and I am actually grateful we didn't catch it sooner. Reminder - we are always right where we are meant to be. And yes, I did say that I am glad we DIDN'T catch it sooner.

When I took time to look back over the symptoms that had accumulated in this time period, with gluten contamination in mind, the picture suddenly became crystal clear. He was no longer the toddler who went GFCF nine years earlier, therefore gluten infractions didn't look quite the same either. With the exception of the school bus incident many years earlier, we really were amateurs at recognizing an infraction with gluten, because we had essentially been feeding him from a dedicated gluten-free environment by making all of his meals at home. There had been no chance of experiencing an infraction.

Since allowing him the freedom to eat out with us more often, his temperament had changed, but it was a slow, insidious evolution. The fact that it didn't strike overnight with a host of new symptoms made it hard to filter out when and how it began. We had been increasingly blaming it on puberty (and don't get me wrong, puberty still had a hand on him, but the waters were muddied by the intro-duction of gluten). His ability to handle the unpredictability of life had regressed excessively, quite similarly to when he was a toddler, except that now his triggers were different. He was increasingly hard to live with, because he was irritable, critical and downright harsh regularly. He found something wrong with everything and was generally negative overall. He had even developed a periodic facial tic once again and we noticed the return of joint inflammation evident by elbow cracking which is something we hadn't seen in years. The burger was the icing on the cake, because it connected the dots for me. It was black and white, he ate a burger willingly out, and then like a scene from a play, drama surrounded the burger we made at home for him.

As you can imagine, this realization was bittersweet. On one hand, we had a solution to a mounting problem, but on the other hand came the (again) painful reminder that food could still be an incredibly destructive force in his life. And the lessons...I'm sure you are wondering what the lessons I speak of are. Well, mine was obvi-ous, I clearly had lost sight of the cues his body was sending us while taking his health for granted.

On a deeper level, it taught me something more valuable, to let go once in a while and follow the guidance of my growing son. You are probably thinking, "Why on earth would you choose to go through such a destructive experience if you could avoid it to begin with?" The simple answer is - for Grayson. The longer answer however holds the magic of the experience. Once we discovered what was going on, I knew that dealing with a 12 year old would be much different than dealing with a 3 or 6 year old. We couldn't just suddenly stop him from eating out like we could when he was three, we needed his participation. I knew I had to help him view this situation in a way that would encourage a vested interest in his health.

So, I did what I do best, I sat him down and spoke with him candidly and from the heart. First, I got his attention by reminding him that for the past few months, he had been expressing distress at the feeling of being out of control emotionally and even physically on occasion. Once I had him on the same page (and agreeing with me) I told him I had discovered the solution. He was cautiously intrigued, but he also knew from experience that discussions like this often resulted in big changes, changes he had no say in.

I started in with an education on the opiate-effect of gluten, dairy and soy, expanding on the details a bit further now that he was older (and it helped me paint the very picture which supported the changes I knew he needed). He instantly saw where this was going when I tied in the fact that "gluten-free" food in a restaurant never comes with any certainties that there won't be cross contamination, and that is because in most places, there usually is, he began slowly shaking his head yes, as the tears accumulated in his eyes. The sign of understanding was precisely this contradiction in pain coupled with awareness. I couldn't hold back my own tears of pain for him. Then, as if we both recognized the lesson together, we turned a corner and released the tension, by bursting out in laughter together.

Just as quickly, he grabbed the reigns back and confidently said, *"I'm going to create a big list of gluten-free dedicated places we can eat"*…then he giggled as he corrected himself, *"I mean, a small list."*

This vested interest in his own health developed purely out of this unexpected gluten challenge. Following our conversation, he (out of habit) continued to ask to eat out with us for a period of time, and a simple reminder was all that was necessary for him to fall back in line with our plan to avoid food that is subject to cross contamination. Looking back, I now know that if we had intervened before Grayson could develop his own sense of awareness, I would have circumvented a major lesson in maturity for him. I consciously knew that at some point, I would need to relinquish control of the boys' health decisions to them, accepting the potential for disruption in their health stability, but this one took me completely by surprise.

WE MUST ALWAYS STAY on our toes and never take our current health status for granted. Even when we have reached what we might consider recovery and things are going smoothly, we must always be alert and open to signs that the body is in distress. It can be so easy to assume that because we've reached a certain plateau of health, that we are safe from the past, but in most cases, we are dealing with genetic mutations that can be turned on and off by our lifestyle choices so getting too relaxed can also cause us to slip backwards again. I will always consider our health to be a vulnerable component of ourselves that requires care and awareness. Our experiences help us build upon our knowledge base allowing us to grow and expand our tools.

23

The shadow truth

THE PROVERBIAL "FINISH LINE"

"The conclusion of a journey is not the end; it is merely the beginning of the next one."

-Dr. Joe Rozencwajg, NMD

WITH THE LIGHT, we must also contend with the shadow, and with recovery must come growing pains. As we embark on this journey to recovery, we have loose ends to tie up, or knot or cut! Although all seems well on the front end, those loose ends prove to have their roots in deep, sometimes even yanking us back a bit. Everyone else sees the recovery angle, our child is no longer Autistic and is past the bulk of his PANDAS symptoms, yes that's a win, two actually, HUGE wins, but it isn't over. Recovery is uneven, it's messy and it's individual.

In our case, the habits that developed throughout the illness period died hard. We had to help our child cultivate the gaps in his development. He appeared to be a healthy, well- balanced pre-teen, but the gaping holes from his past were proving that we had work to do to help him catch up to his peers. I didn't see equalization as our goal, but for his sake, I was sure he was going to want to fit in more and stand out less (for these reasons anyway). Our job had just gotten more interesting, as he was approaching his teens. My perspective is that a parent should guide their child to make their own "good" choices.

How we do that with such large gaps to fill in was yet again, new to us! We have often paved the way in our healing journey, and this was no different.

I was made painfully aware that Grayson would be jumping into a life that he was unfamiliar with, the same kind of life other kids had been actively and developmentally participating in during each and every age and stage of their lives. His social life had been limited by Autism and PANDAS during so many critical years, that he missed out on many valuable life lessons others had already learned years earlier. Learning about acceptable social etiquette is cultivated through hands-on, real-life, age-appropriate experiences. When a young boy who wants so badly to fit in with his peers struggles to identify socially with his peers, it can be a painful lesson for him to handle and maybe even more painful for his family to witness.

It was also hard for most neurotypical kids to comprehend what my child was going through, even his own brother sometimes struggled with what Grayson needed to manage in order to come up to par with his peers. It was frustrating and disheartening for everyone, if we lost sight of the big picture. It was akin to learning how to live life within a completely different culture. We were navigating unchartered waters without a compass. Grayson had to step into many real-life situations for the very first time, much later than his neurotypical counterparts.

Reading body language is often one of the developmental milestones young recovered children lag in. For many who lost eye contact early on, they lost the focus to see and interpret others. For Grayson, this was tricky, because he didn't lose all eye contact and he was quite social, in fact, he leaned more towards over-social without boundaries. In a 10 year old, it looked awkward when he was trying to relate to others his age and they felt he had stepped over boundaries. Kids can be quite cruel inadvertently when they don't understand something.

As a parent who had always protected my vulnerable child, this was new territory for me too, because I felt I must let him take on these experiences head-on in order to fully integrate them into his habitual daily life. If we shelter our children constantly, how can we release them into the world some day? This was the time to let him learn to refine these skills, while we were still there to help soften the blow.

It is during this stage of recovery when we must be aware of the possibility of bullying and as much as I hate to say it, our children aren't always the victims. They can also become the bully, as a defense mechanism. The latter is unfortunately the path Grayson began to follow in order to acquire the results he wanted with his peers. All he knew was that he needed to be strong with others, in order to not be taken advantage of, but with his lack of experience balancing the feelings of others with his own, he fell into the habit of trying to forcefully engage in getting his way. As expected, it resulted in some friction among his friends. With multiple discussions and role playing, we were able to help Grayson manage these situations as they arose.

This is when, as parents, we must respond appropriately and not emotionally, to the incidents. Since he wanted nothing more than to make his friends happy, he jumped at the opportunities to resolve these situations and often did so with enthusiasm and success.

Over time, we discovered that he was managing many situations on his own and his friendships began building in depth and loyalty, which appeared to be lacking in the past.

I feel that we must make the time to help our children by creating opportunities where they can experience hands-on learning. With that in mind, we must also never circumvent some of the painful lessons they inevitably have to endure. As role models, it's even more important to remind ourselves that we must model the behavior we expect from our kids. It's not uncommon to try to prevent children from experiencing adult lessons whether it be about financial hardships, relationships, correcting mistakes or difficult decision making, but by including our children in our lives more fully, we can teach so much!

They see everything anyway, so just because you hide when you have a difficult conversation with someone, doesn't mean they don't feel your energy shift afterwards. How often have you caught yourself responding more negatively to the kids after a stressful situation, in an attempt to "protect" them from what you have just experienced? Instead of protecting them from life, consider inclusion (at an appropriate level they can comprehend) so that they may witness you navigating your own life challenges. This is where the most powerful life lessons occur.

Children often feel that their parents never make mistakes or that they are perfect beings. This inadvertently leads them to believe that they too must be "perfect." No one is perfect, nor should we strive for perfection, but rather balance, compassion and intrinsic happiness. As our children recover, they are going to be more acutely aware of the messages we are subliminally communicating with our own behaviors, which is why I stress the importance of healing our own state of mind.

WHEN OUR CHILDREN reach this stage, there is a misunderstanding that our job as healer is done. Quite the contrary, our role as healer changes shape and takes on a new perspective. The focus shifts. Instead of merely dosing remedies and supplements or managing appointments, we can make an effort to see the world through their eyes so we can customize the remainder of their recovery. Recovery isn't just the cessation of symptoms, it's the merging of all of our worlds more uniformly. Parents, siblings, friends and even strangers hold pertinent pieces to the puzzle, and by bringing it all into focus we shift into the role of becoming our child's life coach. Our children may finally feel good physically, but we are whole beings consisting of a mind, body and spirit. Let's remember to align the whole person in all of our decisions. If we skip over this piece and jump into the depths of life-post-recovery without a life preserver, we may drown.

Don't you wish there was a one-way ticket to recovery, some sort of perfectly designed step-by-step handbook? While there can be right and wrong ways to manage certain healing protocols, some having significant consequences, there is no right or wrong way to navigate recovery for your family. I wish there were a handbook, but even if there were, it wouldn't be perfect for your child, because every person, family and recovery is different…as it should be. Through trial and error, I learned that the only handbook I ever needed was my child's cues. When I finally took the time to tune in to my child, my family and our needs, I had everything I needed right there in front of me. I had to eliminate the noise, which became more challenging as social network groups grew, and opinions, ideas and "magic pills" surfaced day in and day out in these groups. It can be incredibly overwhelming to have too much information and not enough intuition, because you can easily end up chasing multiple paths, becoming derailed frequently.

It is difficult to give preference to any one decision, treatment or lesson when it comes to this stage of our recovery journey, because they all played important roles in the culmination of events that led us to this point. I would say that without a doubt though, choosing to homeschool/unschool our boys was one of the larger chunks in our awakening and I don't mean just for the kids, but for the whole family. I'm aware that this isn't always an option, but I also think you can recreate this lifestyle even with conventional school in place. An unschooling environment is child-led, it encourages freedom to explore life as it comes and it provides the wide open space for learning, for all involved. We have been able to develop stronger relationships with one another by focusing on togetherness in a world where individualism is so highly praised.

. . .

So, was this the end or the beginning? Where did we go from here? Forward! We went forward with all of the lessons behind us and many more on the horizon ahead of us. When we began this journey, I had this ideal in my mind, always picturing "the end"...the end of what? The end of treatments? The end of the diagnosis? The end of our struggles?

With every closed door, a new one opens, but we must be facing forward to notice. This is the beauty of it all, we are free to create our destiny. The only thing that can stand in the way is ourselves. What do you want your life to look like?

I TAKE comfort knowing that homeopathy and a strong belief system will always be there to catch us when we fall. Life will always bring new challenges, choices and lessons. Living a healthy lifestyle and relying on homeopathy is a great foundation, but we must expect to encounter more of the same in our environment. More toxins, more trauma, more triggers. We can't live in bubbles, but what we can do is take each challenge, one at a time, using the tools in our toolbox. So build up that toolbox!

WE CAN RECOVER from dis-ease and we can recover from a chronic negative frame of mind, and always remember the lessons, because they have created who you've become. Are you in control or are you the result of life happening *to* you? I challenge you to pick yourself up off the ground when things get rough. Stand up tall and look forward, because that is the direction life is going. Take control of YOUR life and see the beauty in your potential to manifest whatever is meant to come next. You, and only you, can do that!

PART II

THE RESOURCE GUIDE

Tips for your healing toolbox

"Humanity is now faced with a stark choice. Evolve or die. If the structures of the human mind remain unchanged, we will always end up re-creating the same world, the same evils, the same dysfunction."

-Eckhart Tolle

Throughout the years, we have completely transformed the way we live. Aside from the methods of healing that we chose directly, we were changing little things here and there, reducing toxins in our home and just generally raising the vibration all around us.

Everything carries its own personal vibration. Chemical-laden foods and toxins carry and transmit lower vibrations. Lower vibrations encourage a dis-ease state. Healthy people emit a naturally high vibration. Although at first, we weren't consciously doing this, I realize now that our whole journey included the slow and steady act of raising our vibration collectively in our home (environment), as well as in our bodies. I could probably fill a dozen books with just the details of what we have done to improve our health and well-being while raising our frequencies, but part of each individual journey is to learn where your own path is meant to take you, so it is more important for you to follow your intuition and find what resonates with you.

This Resource Guide contains a list of the more important things that we changed in our environment over time (a long time). Find what resonates with you most and start there. My list is very brief, just to get you started. I would recommend researching anything you find intriguing, so you have all of the information you need to make educated decisions. Some changes are easier and may even be free or inexpensive, while others may require some thought, planning and a good portion of money. Take it in bites you can manage emotionally, physically and/or financially. Know that you will find your magic combination, if you keep reaching for success with an open and positive heart. I think you will find that you will inadvertently begin to align with whatever is most important for your family.

Disclaimer

This is where I must remind you to check with your doctor before trying anything mentioned in my book. The information in this book is not intended or implied to be a substitute for professional medical advice, diagnosis or treatment.

The information provided by Jessica Galligani does not diagnose, prevent, treat or cure illness or disease. Your medical doctor diagnoses and treats medical problems. The information you will receive does not constitute an attempt to practice medicine. If you have medical questions and or emergencies, you should consult your qualified health provider for medical assistance and seek treatment at your nearest emergency facility. Any information provided by Jessica Galligani does not take the place of routine medical care and evaluation by your primary care physician. All content, including text, graphics and information, contained in or available through this book and is not a substitute for medical advice or treatment for specific medical conditions.

Contents

ᒪOXINS

IT HAS BEEN SUGGESTED that children with Autism are the "canaries in the coal mine." This idea stems from the days when coal miners would take canaries into the mines to determine the level of toxicity in the mine, because the canary is sensitive to the carbon monoxide and other gasses and would chirp in warning, become ill or die when exposed to it, giving miners a warning to evacuate. So essentially, the canary in the coal mine is an early warning sign of danger. Likewise, the Autistic population is a sign of an ever-changing evolution of the times, a warning of what is to come.

CHARLES DARWIN UNCOVERED the lengthy process of evolution and how it relates to survival of the fittest, in response to changes in the environment. He found that a single species of bird evolved differently on each of the various small islands of the Galapagos. In order to adapt to its surroundings and survive in accordance with natural selection, each island had a bird from the same species with a beak that was different from the others. The changes in the bird's beak enabled it to find food according to the offerings on that particular island, encouraging survival. This adaptation would then be passed on to its offspring as part of its evolution. Biologist and educator, Regina Bailey, defines evolution as follows:

> "Biological evolution is defined as any genetic change in a population that is inherited over several generations. These changes may be small or large, noticeable or not so noticeable.
>
> In order for an event to be considered an instance of evolution, changes have to occur on the genetic level of a population and be passed on from one generation to the next.
>
> This means that the genes, or more specifically, the alleles in the population change and are passed on. These changes are noticed in the phenotypes (expressed physical traits that can be seen) of the population.

A change on the genetic level of a population is defined as a small-scale change and is called microevolution.

Biological evolution also includes the idea that all of life is connected and can be traced back to one common ancestor. This is called macroevolution. "

HAVE you ever thought about Autism and autoimmune disease as a form of evolution? As our country becomes more toxic, our species needs to adapt to the environment and find ways to either evolve and survive, or we could be looking at a decrease in population.

Many of the deficiencies associated with inherent genetic mutations discovered in the Autism population have been identified as a survival mechanism.

For example, candida overgrowth, which is prominent in Autism, PANDAS/PANS and autoimmune diseases. Candida is able to sequester, or absorb its weight in heavy metals as a means of protecting the body, so is it surprising that those with heavy metal toxicity have elevated levels of candida? We see this as a challenge (much like the symptoms our body produces during the healing phase), because elevated candida comes with obvious consequences on our health, but in a sense, this elevated candida is actually a protective mechanism that our body has developed in response to the environment. If we dig further into the cause of the elevated candida, we will find that the true problem isn't the candida itself, rather it's a symptom of the root problem, which is the increased toxic load that the candida is responding to. If we kill off candida without addressing the cause of the overgrowth, we are then unleashing heavy metals into the bloodstream, which will cause an increase in symptoms, especially if this person has genetic mutations in the methylation pathways. Safe detoxification alone has been known to decrease candida overgrowth.

Now, let's look at autoimmunity as a whole. We've adapted this global theory that an autoimmune condition is a sign that the body is attacking itself, suggesting that nature has gone awry. I don't believe nature goes wrong like this. Evolution has proven time and time again that nature adapts to the conditions of change. So what is autoimmunity, if it isn't a broken immune system? It is adaptation in action! When the body has accumulated toxins or microbes with an affinity for particular organs or tissue, the body's job is to deal with it. We've been told that arthritis is the body attacking its own joints and that PANDAS is the body attacking its own basal ganglia, but I believe that these conditions, like any other systemic response to an invader, are just a more systematic global attempt at the body doing its job.

An infection in the joints, for example, would look like the body is attacking itself, inflammatory markers included, because the joints would be the focal point of the target set by the immune system. When we get a small burn on our finger, inflammation occurs at the site of the damaged tissue in an attempt to heal it, not because the body is attacking its own finger! So, why have we decided that because it's being experienced throughout the body or because the inflammation affects a particular organ system, that the immune system has it all wrong?

Personally, I think autoimmune disease is global inflammation associated with damage done by a toxin and/or a microbe. It's the body mounting a response to an invader, which just happens to also be systemic. The afflicted body tissue is collateral damage in a chronic battle caused by said toxin or microbe. When we view autoimmunity in this way, we can see clearly that the inflammation isn't the root of the problem, it is a manifestation of the problem.

One example of targeting the root cause can be observed through a friend's experience with hypothyroidism, which when left untreated, has been known to progress on to an autoimmune condition known as Hashimoto's, where supposedly the body creates antibodies to attack its own thyroid. When my friend's lab work came back suggesting hypothyroidism, she decided to make an appointment with her Naturopathic Doctor for a second opinion, who chose to scan her thyroid using biofeedback. They discovered that she had the Epstein Barr Virus (EBV) in her thyroid. She was told to apply Thieve's essential oil topically to her thyroid once per day. Low and behold, her next set of labs were normal. This is an example of a condition that was set in motion by a virus. Over time, without treatment, the body would have amped up its immune response and may have even begun trying to attack the virus in her thyroid.

Could this have looked a lot like Hashimoto's, with the body developing antibodies to its own organ, as a way to target the location? And may she have also had elevated EBV titers, had the mainstream doctor known to look for this virus in connection with her thyroid symptoms? Who knows, but what we do know is that her hypothyroid condition was reversed by simply and naturally addressing the infection. We also know that if she had chosen to use a conventional endocrinologist, she would have likely been put on Synthroid (a synthetic thyroid medication that increases T4) and what would that have done for the infection in her thyroid? Absolutely nothing. The EBV would have continued to inhabit her thyroid, encouraging more damage, which may have eventually become Hashimoto's. Hashimoto's is an autoimmune thyroid disorder typified by the immune system attacking its own thyroid. When the thyroid becomes the target of the immune system's activation we can imagine that something has instigated a chronic response by the immune system within the thyroid, in this case the EBV.

It is evident through even just these two scenarios that evolution has taken place and although we don't necessarily like the results, our bodies are in fact trying to manage the damage done by society. How do we heal from these types of toxicities? We need to reduce the toxic load and increase our capacity for natural detoxification.

Sadly, toxicities are at an all-time high, so naturally, reproduction may begin to spiral downward in response to this, which is ultimately a global experiment in survival of the fittest. A study has recently also confirmed that this is the first generation which will live shorter lives than their parent's generation.

HERE IS A VERY basic presentation of how toxins effect our bodies. First, you must understand what a toxin is. Toxins consist of anything that the body cannot metabolize or anything that is foreign to the body. Sources of toxins are: food, water, noise, dramatic changes in weather, EMFs causing excessive radiation, emotional trauma, even an excess of normal chemicals in the body, and meta-toxins which are the result of metabolized foods that cannot be eliminated. It is a commonly known fact that our bodies are 70% water. However, in actuality, that number is greater. I learned during a lecture by Dr. Robyn Murphy, ND that 99.5% of all molecules in the body are water. One molecule of a toxin (nicotine, stress hormone, GMO foods, etc.) will lock up 1000 molecules of water in our cell. That cell will begin to die or mutate, then it stops functioning. Once 20-30% of an organ's cellular function is down, you start seeing disease. The degeneration of intracellular fluids is the basis of all diseases.

DETOXIFICATION IS at the heart of just about every recovery, from multiple diseases. I love the way Ellen Kamhi, PhD, RN also known as the "Natural Nurse" once said it, *"Pharmaceuticals do nothing but suppress the symptoms. If you want to stop the break down process [inflammation] you need to do detoxification."* When our bodies can't detoxify effectively enough, we store these toxins (in fat cells, tissues, organs and bones) which is a safety mechanism designed by the body, unfortunately this also means we are harboring them until we do something to encourage the body to release them.

There are two parts to the process of managing detoxification and both are necessary to see success in management of toxins. First, we must reduce the intake of toxins from our environment and second, we must help our bodies release and effectively remove the toxins they are holding on to. This can be tricky if you have genetic mutations in your methylation pathways, causing bottle-necking of these toxins as they try to leave the body.

This will result in an uptick in symptoms, meaning the detox organs are being strained. So, caution and balance must always be a top priority in your choices.

The more you know about your genetic make-up, the better off you will be in deciding which detox methods and supplements work best for your family. And remember, this is purely the physical aspect of recovery, which is only one part of the full picture. Even though we have tried many different means of detoxifying, I would rate the top contenders to be: far infrared sauna, IonCleanse foot bath and the Spooky 2 rife machine combined with BioPure Chlorella Growth Factor, cilantro tincture, and binders like BioPure ZeoBind, Advanced TRS or Activated Charcoal. Regardless of your detox choices, supporting your organs is a must.

"Toxemia is not the cause of all disease. HOW you got toxic is the cause of all disease." -Dr. Robyn Murphy, ND.

WHILE I BELIEVE it is important to detoxify our lives, our environments and our bodies, which is what this section of the resource guide is all about, the all too true statement above from Dr. Murphy reminds us that we must also consider that our susceptibilities set the stage for how our bodies will handle the variety of toxins thrown at us from the environment. Exploring modalities that encourage you to peel back the layers of what led you down the path you are on, from conception, may prove to be incredibly helpful and even preventative. I personally feel that homeopathy has this amazing ability to peel back these layers successfully, but don't stop there, because I'm sure there are many potential treatments that fit the definition of inherent soul work.

On the physical plane, unnecessary gadgets aimed at making life easier often introduce toxins into our world and lives. The easy button has created a monster, both financially and morally, and our world, in its entirety, is suffering far-reaching consequences to this and future generations. So please, always consider the next seven generations in your decisions.

AIR PURIFIERS

Depending on the environment, it's often helpful for those who are sensitive to have a good air purifier running regularly. We tried a few, but liked one that combined hospital grade HEPA filteration with UV light to control microbes in the air. We found this especially helpful after remediation for mold in our home. At minimum, it gave me the peace of mind I needed to stop worrying about the quality of the air in our home. Be sure to find one that doesn't recirculate toxins or worse, add to them. There are many wonderful and effective brands out there now.

There are also great PCO (Photocatalytic Oxidation) and PECO (Photo Electrochemical Oxidation) products available for safely and effectively disinfecting the air without leaving behind dangerous mycotoxins. PECO and PCO air purifiers will literally break down toxins (including mold and it's mycotoxins) at a molecular level. The differences you will find in the technology will most likely lead you to choose one style or the other.

Active PCO units will send hydroxyl free radicals into the air where they will hunt down toxins like mold spores, mycotoxins, pollen, dander, viruses, VOCs (volatile organic compounds), formaldehyde, ozone and other toxins. The hydroxyl molecules only survive a few seconds before they bind with the toxins in the air and on surfaces, then they break down the molecules into harmless molecules normally found in the air. PECO units are passive and will only treat the air that passes through the air purifier and may be more tolerable for extra sensitive individuals. When either of these types of air purifiers are initially introduced into an environment, it's a good idea to let them run in an unoccupied area until the toxin contamination is reduced. Intolerance tends to correlate with the amount of toxins being broken down in the air which suggests that there is a sensitivity to the decomposition process of these molecules for some people.

We reacted near our PCO unit during the first few weeks of decontamination so we made a habit of opening windows briefly every now and then to air out the space, but leaving them open for too long in contaminated locations, can slow down the decontamination process. Leaving the units on only when you sleep is another method of decontaminating without irritating all of the inhabitants of the house. Again though, it will take longer to get through the initial clean-up phase, but it will be much more tolerable and gentle, so if you need to do this for someone who is sensitive in the house, don't even think twice. We chose to treat areas we weren't spending time in while we were awake and then we treated the areas we spend the most time in during our days, at night when we were sleeping. Once we were past the initial decontamination phase, we could tolerate the units as if they weren't even there.

They tend to have an odor only when they are breaking down mold and VOCs, and our reaction period directly correlated to these odors. When you notice a burning smell, it is likely that the hydroxyls have found and are decomposing mold. A more chemical odor is most likely the decomposition of VOCs. I remember when we put our units on the second floor of our home, where we have wall to wall carpeting (I know, this is a project for another day, it isn't ideal), the odor was completely different from the odor we noticed downstairs. It reminded me of opening up a new plastic doll as a child. As we move our units around the house, sometimes there is a faint odor for a few hours as the unit clears up areas that weren't as easily accessible to the original decontamination phase.

We have a small 1920's beach bungalow in my home state where we spend our summers and using a PCO (HiTech, in particular) was life changing for us! For the first few summers that we owned the home, we were struggling with regression in both boys, and I personally felt angry and anxious while we were there. I was having ear pain on and off as well, so I knew the signs. Considering it was a vacation home and we loved being there, our moods should have been excitement, elation and joy, rather than anger, impatience, and irritation. It quickly became clear to me that we were dealing with mold.

Since we couldn't remediate right away, because there was no sure fire way to establish where the mold was coming from, we tried all kinds of things to help our bodies detox it faster like: chlorella, cilantro and ZeoBind paired with IonCleanse foot baths. I tried everything I could think of to address the mold in the air, I used essential oil diffusers, bee propolis diffusers, timed probiotic aerosol sprayers, I even fogged with an environmental probiotic spray, and while some things provided a bit of relief, nothing completely eliminated the agitation brewing through the house every summer. I even tried the highly acclaimed PECO called Molekule. As long as it was on its highest (and loudest setting) it provided some relief, but it just wasn't enough.

We came to the disappointing conclusion that we might have to sell our vacation home, the very home that brought us closer to my family, the children's cousins and the ocean. The grounding opportunities provided by the ocean was so healing, and being near family was incredibly fulfilling and joyful. We looked forward to spending this quality time with relatives that we would otherwise only see once a year. This was devastating. I decided to give it one last ditch effort.

Because the HiTech is so expensive I was really holding out on this idea, but selling our home and dumping all the beautiful things we had filled it with was much more expensive and emotional, so we made the investment and put a couple thousand dollars into the technology that NASA deemed safe for their astronauts and hospitals used in neonatal units. I felt justified in the expense and the experiment, because the alternative was just too painful.

We did HERTSMI testing (a scoring system for water damaged buildings) to confirm that in just four short weeks, our score went from an 18 (considered dangerous) to a 4 (well under safe)!! All we did was deploy one HiTech (each covers 1600 square feet of living space) and I cleaned with an environmental probiotic one week before taking our dust samples.

Immediately following the decontamination phase, we all began to feel more like ourselves, growing more balanced every day. We were able to salvage our summers without the drastic step of selling everything! It was not a long term solution, but it certainly bought us more time to figure out what we wanted to do going forward. It also meant that if we decided to buy a different beach house, we could take our belongings without fear of cross contamination.

Beach houses are in humid environments, and it would be naive of me to think we can completely eliminate all mold, so HiTech was an invaluable tool for us to maintain this great joy in our lives, without contributing to ill health in our family. We now own two units for our primary home and one for the beach house. They are on 24/7 and we feel great in our safe spaces. They can be used to decontaminate moldy cars as well.

We used ours to eliminate severe nicotine odors in my father's truck. He was a chain smoker, and his truck was so bad that there was nicotine caked on everything. After steam cleaning to get it out of the fabric and then running the HiTech in his truck for about 5 days, the odor was eliminated. We did end up running it for a few more days after the heat of the spring released a little more into the cab. I couldn't tolerate even a few minutes in the cab before using the HiTech in it. I would immediately start creating mucus in my throat, my eyes would hurt and I would feel foggy headed. This technology proved to be nothing short of amazing.

Taking it one step further, there are also units that can be installed directly into the air duct vents for more effective distribution. This sounds enticing, but should also be conducted only with sufficient evidence that the product being used (and distributed throughout your home) is one everyone will tolerate. When we had to replace our HVAC and air conditioning, we decided on adding an electrostatic filter and a UV lamp to cut down on toxins running through our vents, as an added precaution. Then we added a few different types of stand-alone air purifiers since we like to change our plans frequently, based on new technology and information. Do your research, your time will be well spent in this arena.

ALUMINUM

Avoid it. Aluminum foil, aluminum cans, aluminum pots, pans and cookie sheets. Aluminum in baking soda. Aluminum in deodorant. And my favorite, aluminum being injected into our children with every vaccination. Even the CDC has made statements on their website about aluminum that elude to its toxicity, such as

> "*People exposed to high levels of aluminum may develop Alzheimer's disease*" and "*Very young animals appeared weaker and less active in their cages and some movements appeared less coordinated when their mothers were exposed to large amounts of aluminum during pregnancy and while nursing. In addition, aluminum also affected the animal's memory. These effects are similar to those that have been seen in adults. Brain and bone disease caused by high levels of aluminum in the body have been seen in children with kidney disease. Bone disease has also been seen in children taking some medicines containing aluminum. In these children, the bone damage is caused by aluminum in the stomach preventing the absorption of phosphate, a chemical compound required for healthy bones.*"[1]

How is it then that they approve of and support the use of aluminum in children's vaccinations, at doses that are higher than the EPA drinking water standards which are . 05-.2mg/L (milligrams per liter)? The amount of aluminum in the DTaP is .33-.625mg per dose, the Hib vaccine has .225mg per dose, the Hep A .225-.25mg per dose, the combined DTaP/polio/HepB vaccine has a whopping .85mg per dose, the HPV vaccine has .5mg per dose. Do the math as you begin to combine vaccinations. By the time a child is 18-months-old, they have received the equivalence of about 4-5mg of injectable aluminum from their vaccinations. Aluminum does not belong in the body, it's a heavy metal with dire consequences, including Autism, ADHD, cancers, dementia, MS and Alzheimer's Disease. Heavy metals bioaccumulate in our bones, tissues and organs.

Aluminum can migrate into your food from cookware, utensils and aluminum foil. Chemical Engineer and researcher at the American University of Sharjah, Dr. Essam Zubaidy, found that cooking with aluminum foil leaches *over* 400mg of aluminum into your food, especially while cooking vegetables such as tomatoes, citrus juices and spices. The higher the temperature, the more the aluminum leaches, emitting parts of the metal into the food. Every time you cook with aluminum foil, imagine you are popping a capsule with 400mg of aluminum into your mouth! Now, imagine doing that every time you cook with aluminum foil! Considering aluminum has an accumulative effect on the body and brain, there is a good chance that much of this aluminum is being stored rather than excreted.

Robert F. Kennedy, Jr. of the Children's Health Defense noted:

> *Dr. Christopher Exley's study is on aluminum in the brains of 10 donors who had Autism. They contained some of the highest levels of aluminum ever recorded in human brain, and the aluminum was found in the brain's immune cells, the microglia and the cells which provide support and protection for the neurons, the glia. How does a 15 year old have as much aluminum in his brain as someone who is many decades older who has died of familial Alzheimer's disease? Dr. Exley's findings have shocking implications for today's generation of children who receive 5,000 mcg. of aluminum in vaccines by the age of 18 months and up to 5,250 additional mcg if all recommended boosters, HPV and meningitis vaccines are administered.* [2]

---

1. Agency for Toxic Substances and Diseases Registry, "Public Health Statement for Aluminum" (Sept. 2008). https://www.atsdr.cdc.gov/phs/phs.asp?id=1076&tid=34
2. Children's Health Defense: High Aluminum Found in Autism Brain Tissue (Nov. 2017) https://childrenshealthdefense.org/news/high-aluminum-found-autism-brain-tissue/

CASTOR OIL PACKS FOR THE LIVER

The liver is responsible for over 500 biochemical functions in the body, some of which are: metabolism of fats, proteins and carbohydrates, storage of vitamins, minerals and sugars, blood filtration which removes chemicals and bacteria, storage of extra blood which can be released as needed, breaks down and eliminates excess hormones, helps regulate electrolyte and water balance, creates immune substances, detoxification of drugs and noxious substances. Signs of a sluggish liver can be: unrefreshed sleep, yellowish hue to the whites of the eyes and/or skin, a yellow or mapped tongue, teeth marks in the sides of the tongue, chemical sensitivities, frequent headaches related to tension or eye strain, skin problems such as rashes, psoriasis, acne and dry or oily skin, brittle nails, weak tendons, ligaments, and muscles, restlessness from 11pm to 2am, impatience, anger, frustrating easily, blocked creativity and tendency to bruise easily.

Castor oil is extracted from the seed of the Ricininus communis which is rich in ricineoleic acid and only exists in castor oil. Double blind studies by the Association for Research and Enlightenment, Inc. demonstrated that castor oil packs increase T-cells originating from bone marrow and the thymus gland which are used to destroy invaders like bacteria, fungi and viruses. It also has the ability to increase liver activity, improve digestion, increase lymphatic flow and balance the nervous system. For children who won't sit still for a castor oil pack, you can rub some into the torso, near the liver, before bed and put an old shirt on (to avoid staining a good shirt).

CHLORELLA

There was a time when I was a die-hard follower of the late Andrew Cutler low-dose, oral chelation protocol and that requires dogmatic views about his beliefs. He was undeniably a brilliant man, a pioneer in his field, but had me believing that the *only* way to remove metals from the body was through his method. The only problem with this is it used fear tactics to support his theory. There was suggestion that he had done all the research to prove anything else only mobilizes the metals, not eliminating them. I was literally afraid to touch anything else for years! When I stopped allowing fear to make decisions for me, I began paying attention to families, scientists and doctors who were seeing progress using other methods of slow gentle detoxification of a natural form.

I eventually researched this avenue more and began to experiment very slowly and cautiously. At first, chlorella threw us all over the edge. It would make us incredibly irritable, sensitive and tired, suggesting our livers weren't handling the detox well, aka - toxic overload. So as you can imagine, this would cause pause and I would fall back into the pattern of, "Cutler said it was dangerous, it must be!" It went on like this for a while, I would try it, back off, try it, back off, always out of fear that I could be causing more harm than good. Eventually, I felt like we needed to detox more than just metals, so I dug into the research of chlorella again and came to the conclusion that we needed to consider it to help open our detox pathways. Chlorella fit the bill in so many ways.

When I learned that chlorella also detoxifies radiation, pesticides and herbicides in addition to heavy metals while improving nutrition exponentially, I decided to give it a try again. In combination with an IonCleanse foot bath and eventually a far infrared sauna, we were able to tolerate liquid Chlorella Growth Factor from BioPure. It is the brand recommended by Dr. Dietrich Klinghardt, a pioneer in lyme and mold recovery, both of which are often entangled in our Autism and PANDAS/PANS webs.

I was ready to listen to and trust someone else finally, and it began to show promise. Once we had incorporated safer ways to open up more detox pathways, we began (at different paces) handling the chlorella, but only that type initially. Regardless of what type of chlorella you choose to try, be sure it is broken-cell wall chlorella. We even began to see rapid growth of both boys each time we tried the liquid Chlorella Growth Factor. To bring out the best in chlorella, pair it with cilantro, which has the unique ability to liberate toxins from the brain. The cilantro loosens the toxins and chlorella binds with them ensuring that they leave the body. I also took Dr. Klinghardt's advice on using a binder known as ZeoBind from BioPure to be sure we weren't letting any toxins escape their demise. Citrus pectin is another well-known effective binder. So as you can see, using chlorella isn't something you can experiment with in a vacuum, meaning it requires other supports and an open detox pathway to function optimally.

We now take chlorella and cilantro at higher doses with ease...and results! But be aware that it took us many months of using super small amounts along with, at minimum, an IonCleanse foot bath. That is only our experience, and I wouldn't suggest this will definitely work for everyone, but it's something to discuss with your doctor, if you have trouble tolerating chlorella of any kind. Please research your chlorella sources extensively since many products have been found to be tainted with heavy metals, and clearly using a product with high heavy metals would be counterproductive.

**CAUTION - do not disrupt heavy metals in the body using products like chlorella, cilantro or any other "chelator" if you currently have amalgam fillings in your mouth.

See more about chlorella in "Nutrition."

COOKING OILS

Perhaps you didn't expect to see cooking oils under the heading of "toxins," but what you might not realize is that even healthy oils can become incredibly unhealthy, if they are heated to a temperature that exceeds their smoking point, the heat quickly turns the oil rancid and rancid oils provoke free radicals in the body. Free radicals are a cause of cancer, so in essence, cooking oils heated beyond their smoke point become carcinogenic. An alternative to heating your oils is to use them after the food is cooked, as a drizzle on top, as you serve the food. I know, some foods just need that extra crunch a good cooking oil produces, so knowing the smoke point of healthy oils is a must! You will notice from the list below that the refined oils tend to have higher smoke points, but the trade-off also means that the refined oils have been hit with processing and heat treatments that might have already decimated the Omega-3 content.

Try to keep the balance of Omega-6 to Omega-3 fatty acids in mind when choosing your oils. Omegas 6 and 3 are essential to health, but a diet too high in Omega-6 can prevent the body from properly metabolizing Omega-3. More importantly, Omega-6 from vegetable oils in particular, is known to create inflammation. Choosing an oil with a 1:1 Omega 6 to 3 ratio and a medium to high smoke point means that heating the oil won't destroy it's omega-3 content. The number in parentheses below, is the Omega 6 to 3 ratio.

- Unrefined sunflower oil (40:1) - 225°F/107°C
- Unrefined high-oleic sunflower oil (40:1) - 320°F/160°C Extra virgin olive oil (10:1) (high in Omega-9) - 320°F/160°C
- Unrefined walnut oil (5:1) - 320°F/160°C Hemp seed oil (3:1) - 330°F/165°C Butter (9:1) - 350°F/177°C
- Coconut oil (88:1) (contains 66% medium chain

triglycerides) - 350°F/177°C Unrefined sesame oil (138:1) - 350°F/177°C

- Macadamia nut oil (1:1) - 390°F/199°C Semi-refined walnut oil (5:1) - 400°F/204°C
- High quality (low acidity) extra virgin olive oil (13:1) - 405°F/207°C Sesame oil (42:1) - 410°F/210°C
- Grapeseed oil (676:1) - 420°F/216°C Virgin olive oil (13:1) - 420°F/216°C Almond oil (Omega-6 only) - 420°F/216°C
- Hazelnut oil (no Omega-3, 78% Omega-9) - 430°F/221°C Sunflower oil (40:1) - 440°F/227°C
- Refined high-oleic sunflower oil (39:1) - 450°F/232°C Semi-refined sesame oil (138:1) - 450°F/232°C
- Semi-refined sunflower oil (40:1) - 450°F/232°C Extra light olive oil (High in Omega-9) - 468°F/242°C Ghee (clarified butter) (0:0) - 485°F/252°C
- Avocado oil (12:1) - 520°F/271°C

DENTAL HEALTH

Any good recovery plan must include the exploration of dental contributions. Heavy metals and cavitation sites will significantly impact overall health and are often overlooked. Did you know that "silver" amalgam fillings are actually 50% mercury by weight, and that this mercury (and the array of other metals) is released by the simple act of chewing, heat from food and drink and EMF exposure like cell phone use? According to Dr. Dietrich Klinghardt, one cell phone call can liberate 600 times more mercury from your amalgam fillings! What many don't realize is that mercury toxicity is generational being passed down from our grandmothers, to our mothers and then to us in utero. We are actually born with mercury even before we are exposed to our own sources, of which there are many. According to Dr. Daniel Pompa, it's been confirmed by biopsy that the number of fillings in a pregnant woman's mouth is directly proportionate to the mercury in the baby's brain. It was mentioned in the study "Environmental Mercury and Its Toxic Effects" by Kevin M. Rice, Ernest M. Walker, Jr, Miaozong Wu, Chris Gillette, and Eric R. Blough, that the estimated half-life of mercury in the brain can be as long as 20 years.[1]

The International Academy of Oral Medicine and Toxicology has publicly shared information about the hazards of mercury in amalgam fillings:

> *"Mercury vapor is continuously emitted from dental amalgam fillings, and much of this mercury is absorbed and retained in the body. The output of mercury can be intensified by the number of fillings and other activities, such as chewing, teeth-grinding, and the consumption of hot liquids. Mercury is also known to be released during the placement, replacement, and removal of dental amalgam fillings.*
>
> *One reason for the wide range of symptoms is that mercury taken into the body can accumulate in virtually any organ. An estimated 80% of the mercury vapor from dental amalgam fillings is absorbed by the*

lungs and passed to the rest of the body, particularly the brain, kidney, liver, lung, and gastrointestinal tract. The half life of metallic mercury varies depending on the organ where the mercury was deposited and the state of oxidation, and mercury deposited in the brain can have a half life of up to several decades. Toxic effects of this mercury exposure vary by individual, and one or a combination of symptoms can be present and can change over time. An array of co-existing factors influence this personalized reaction to dental mercury including the presence of other health conditions, the number of amalgam fillings in the mouth, gender, genetic predisposition, dental plaque, exposure to lead, consumption of milk, alcohol, or fish, and more.

In addition to the fact that individual response to mercury varies, the effects of these exposures are even more insidious because it can take many years for symptoms of mercury poisoning to manifest themselves, and previous exposures, especially if they are relatively low-level and chronic (as is often the case from dental amalgam fillings), might not be associated with the delayed onset of symptoms. It is not surprising that just as there are a wide range of mercury poisoning symptoms, there are also a wide range of health risks related to dental amalgam fillings."

Dental revision should be done only by a qualified mercury-free or biological dentist who uses the strictest prevention methods and I would recommend looking into Huggins licensed professionals if you would like to take your safety a step further. A Huggins trained dentist will also consider the electrical charge emitted by the filling(s) and only removes them in a particular order that is conducive to healing rather than degeneration and autoimmunity.

A cavitation brings a completely different health challenge to the surface in terms of how dental health can influence the health of the body. A cavitation, which is a hole in the bone, usually where a tooth had been extracted in the past, can actually occur anywhere in the body, but is most often found in the jawbones. Jawbone cavitations often host silent infections that have the capacity to leave the site of the bone and enter the blood stream causing a variety of symptoms and has even been linked to cancer. Dr. Boyd Haley, the head of Chemistry at the University of Kentucky has shown that the toxins from cavitation to be more potent than botulinum toxin! A knowledgeable biological dentist can clean out these dangerous cesspools with ozone, preventing further damage.

In my own personal experience with a full dental revision involving 8 amalgam fillings and 4 cavitation sites, I immediately experienced resolution to foot neuralgia I had been experiencing for years. It went away literally overnight. I have heard about miraculous recoveries from MS, neurological disorders, memory loss, anger, anxiety, tinnitus and more. Don't overlook this hidden health hazard!

---

1. K.M. Rice, E.M. Walker, Jr, M. Wu, C. Gillette, E.R. Blough. *Environmental Mercury and Its Toxic Effects*. Journal of Preventative Medicine & Public Health (Mar. 2014); 47(2): 74-83. Published online 2014 Mar 31. doi: 10.3961/jpmph.2014.47.2.74

DETOX TONIC

This is a method of homeopathic detoxification introduced to me by Dr. Robyn Murphy during my years as a homeopathic student. It is a brilliant way to fine tune the detoxification process of specific things you want to address. Using a large (12+ ounce) bottle of spring water, you add a cell salt (or two) of choice, an herb of choice and a homeopathic remedy to address the toxin you want to detox. In clinical trials where this was done with heavy metal remedies like mercury and aluminum, the corresponding metals were subsequently elevated in urine samples. I would caution you not to do this with a heavy metal remedy if you have amalgam fillings in your mouth.

An example of how we use this method would be when we are exposed to mold. I use a few pellets of Bioplasma cell salts, a squirt of cilantro tincture and some chlorella and a homeopathic mold nosode 30C potency. Give the bottle about ten shakes and then either drink the whole thing before 11am to use it as a flush or you can sip the water throughout the day. Do this for about a week and then re-evaluate. I like to do this with homeopathic glyphosate periodically just to be sure we are eliminating glyphosate regularly. I also follow up with a dose of ZeoBind (a powdered zeolite product by BioPure) about an hour after I finish my detox tonic, to bind with any stray toxins.

ENEMA

There is an interesting stigma to the discussion of enemas. Most of us aren't learning about them from our family because for some reason putting something into the rectum is taboo and embarrassing. Well, I'm here to tell you that if you haven't tried an enema yet, you really should consider it! Enemas are a form of hygiene that can't be duplicated any other way. We wash our hair to remove build up, soap up our bodies to remove toxins from our skin, we brush our teeth to reduce pathogenic microbes, cotton swabs and ear candling cleans the ear canals and neti pots to clean out nasal cavities. We can also cleanse our bowels and there is no better way to aid in more effective detoxification of the bowels then to do a quick enema.

Some of the great reasons to use enemas:

- Constipation and/or diarrhea, even acutely
- Have trouble detoxing
- Have been using a detoxification modality and you want to support elimination
- Dehydration
- Sickness that prevents you from keeping fluids down (this is a great way to avoid going to the ER for fluids, but research the solution mixture you want to use for rehydration, because it requires some salt in your enema water, in fact, all enemas should have a little saline in them so they don't suck minerals from your bowels)
- Skin problems
- Chronic headaches
- Allergies
- Fatigue
- Depression
- Back pain
- Sinus problems

- Indigestion
- Inoculate your bowels with a probiotic, herb or minerals directly

If you are experiencing die off from a detoxification regimen or you are experiencing symptoms of bowel disorder for any reason, an enema is a quick way to release toxins that have the potential to ferment in the bowels, causing the recirculation of neurotoxins.

Metatoxins that have been processed by the body for elimination are actually more toxic, and combined with slow elimination, can be detrimental causing symptoms as they remain backed up in the intestines. If you are not experiencing 2-3 bowel movements per day, it is likely that you are already backed up. Surprisingly, most cases of chronic diarrhea actually stem from compacted bowels.

My grandmother was old school and she openly discussed enemas in our household, but I didn't try one until I was in my 40's! Yep, I was one of those resistant parties at one time too. It just sounded frightening to me, but when I realized that we really needed to help our bodies eliminate the metatoxins from our stringent detoxification regimen, I decided it was time to face my fears. What I discovered was that there was nothing to fear! Grandma was right! Using the right supplies aids in a gentle, liberating and rejuvenating experience! And the immediate energy and clarity that I felt afterwards was addictive!

We use an enema bucket from Joe Ball Company with tiny silicone enema catheters which are practically undetectable when inserted with a lubricating oil like coconut oil. Always make sure your water is boiled (to kill pathogens) and cooled to lukewarm so it doesn't shock your system and create an uncomfortable sensation which will force you to evacuate sooner than you should. Expect the first few times to be your experimentation enemas, because the new sensation of liquid rising in your lower intestines will trigger you to release faster than anticipated, so you will use less liquid the first few times, as a result. With practice, you will find yourself holding more liquids and for longer durations.

When we were doing this with our kids, we encouraged them to lie on the bathroom floor with a towel under their body, a pillow under their head and I would let them play with a handheld video game for distraction. Since we don't allow electronics often, it was an easy sell! Expect the first enema to be messy, just expect it! It's likely that as soon as they feel the water, they will want to stand up and run to the toilet…or, they may not even stand up and run. Yeah, like I said, it can be messy. Our first experience proved to me that our son didn't know he would have to hold in the fluids, so make sure they know what to expect. You may even want the first one to be experienced in a bathtub. It's important to stay positive and not express any of your own inhibitions when administering the enema, or your child will pick up on that and they will be resistant. They read us like books, they know when we are hesitant or worried, so center yourself BEFORE you attempt to administer the first enema.

It is our job as their parents to model important hygiene practices and this would be no exception. If your children are young enough, they can sit in with you while you do your own (talking through the process and feelings) or if they are older, you can announce when you are going to do your own enema. It's essential that we pass on healthy hygienic practices like brushing our teeth and taking showers. If you only do enemas on your child and you never conduct them on yourselves, they will also pick up on that.

So what are you waiting for, go to joeballcompany.com for your supplies (or anywhere that carries stainless steel enema buckets) and get started, you will thank me!

Note - be aware that an enema should only be inserted a few inches into the rectum.

FAR INFRARED (FIR) SAUNA

Your skin is a major detoxification organ, but many people don't sweat on a regular basis. I can't speak highly enough about the benefits experienced by FIR saunas. The level of detoxification obtained by regular use is unmatched. I know this is probably the most costly item on the list, but it is not completely unattainable either, so don't write it off just yet. Many wellness centers also have them, and you can pay per session. A one-person sauna can fit easily into an average sized room because it is about the size of a closet and since it is dry heat, there is no risk of moisture accumulation. If there is anything I would recommend starting a savings fund for, it's this!

You must, however, balance your desire for a sauna with safety. There are a lot of cheap saunas out there and you might be tempted to save a few bucks to acquire one sooner, but these saunas are dangerous and counterproductive due to the off-gassing of toxins like adhesives and varnishes. You also want to be sure the wood it's made from is kiln dried and doesn't release any of its own toxins.

Another consideration is Electromagnetic Frequency (EMF) exposure. Some brands take this very seriously and invest a lot of time and money into addressing this growing concern, while others do not. While the seats in many units have low or even zero EMF, the wall readings vary depending on where the wiring is running and you would also want to be sure to test all the different types Electromagnetic Radiation (EMR). Body voltage would indicate the effects the EMR has on the body while sitting in a sauna. We don't lean against the walls, we lean on a backrest which is an optional accessory. It props us away from the wall while adding comfort.

I like to use my sauna time to meditate and clear my mind. I always do it first thing in the morning after a big glass of water, I turn on my calm meditation music and close the door. It's a great way to start the day, especially after some form of workout. Since you will sweat profusely, you will also lose electrolytes so it is important to remain hydrated and replace electrolytes. I like to coordinate our doses of chlorella, cilantro and an effective binder around sauna use. Dr. Dietrich Klinghardt said that using a sauna without these things will displace toxins from "one compartment to another," meaning it can cause redistribution without some support.

Another very important detail he stresses about sauna detoxification is that you MUST wipe off your sweat immediately as you are experiencing it, because toxins are fat soluble and they will sit on your skin. If you wait until you leave the sauna and go to the shower to rinse off, the toxins sitting on the surface on the skin have already reabsorbed into the body. A little knowledge goes a long way.

Now, for some facts about how saunas work. FIR saunas use infrared light, which is the same healing energy that is released by the sun, to heat the body from within, unlike traditional saunas which heat the air like an oven. It is for this reason that FIR saunas are more effective at lower, more tolerable temperatures (130 vs. 200+ degrees) than traditional saunas. Sweat from a FIR experience is composed of 80-85% water, the rest being composed of cholesterol, fat-soluble toxins, heavy metals, sulfuric acid, ammonia, sodium and uric acid (and this last one is music to my ears, because of our oxalate accumulation tendencies). It has also been noted that calcium is excreted during a FIR sauna, but not the usable calcium the body needs, but toxic synthetic calcium that the body can't utilize. The sweat from a traditional sauna is composed of approximately 95-97% water, which means only 5-3% is true detoxification by comparison to 15-20% with the FIR sauna. So, as you can see, sweating can help reduce your toxic load.

This isn't all the FIR sauna is good for. Elevating body temperature, even just slightly, kills viruses and other microbes, including cancer cells. FIR saunas are ideal for mold toxicity recovery! For those with methylation issues, a FIR sauna should be at the top of your list, because releasing toxins via the pathway of the skin reduces the burden on the organs. In many European Countries, saunas are as commonplace and as essential as bathrooms, I would love to see a FIR sauna in every American home! Perhaps than we wouldn't be one of the sickest industrialized Nations on the planet.

GLYPHOSATE

Glyphosate is essentially an antibiotic, killing off beneficial bacteria, resulting in an overgrowth of bad bacteria, promoting inflammation. This overgrowth has been linked to cancers like colorectal, stomach and gallbladder cancers, as well as lymphoma. The overgrowth of bad bacteria results in an endotoxin known as Zonulin, which promotes leaky gut as well as leaky brain. Undigested proteins in the brain result in autoimmune disease. When glyphosate was originally patented in 1964, it was meant to be a chelator of trace minerals, magnesium especially, which has been shown to be another probable cause of cancer.

Our beneficial bacteria use something known as the Shikimic-acid pathway to produce essential nutrients like folate and aromatic amino acids that our bodies can't make. These amino acids are precursors to all kinds of biologically active molecules in our body.

Glyphosate blocks the Shikimate pathway. Promoters of glyphosate debate that there are no ill effects to humans, because we don't have a Shikimate pathway, but the residents of our microbiome do and they are essential to our lives.

One of the most troubling concerns associated with ingesting glyphosate is that it is a synthetic amino acid and glycine analog which can become incorporated into proteins in place of glycine. What does this mean? It means that glyphosate is pretending to be glycine. There is a code for glycine and because glyphosate looks just like glycine, it gets picked up. It fits right into the glycine socket perfectly. Glyphosate then gets in the way, disrupting enzyme function, therefore the proper enzymatic reactions won't happen, in other words, these functions become non-operative. Glycine is normally used in DNA and RNA transcription, protein and enzyme synthesis and collagen formation.

"An amino acid analog of glycine clobbers all life. Glyphosate is the only glycine analog that exists." -Dr. Stephanie Seneff

An overview of the potential harmful effects glyphosate is responsible for, according to research conducted by Dr. Stephanie Seneff of MIT:[12]

- It is a synthetic glycine analog, allowing it to get into proteins
- DNA/RNA dysregulation which ultimately disrupts mitochondrial function and ATP production
- Interferes with the sulfation pathway which is essential for excreting toxins like aluminum, mercury and xenobiotics
- Disruption of sulfate synthesis and transport also impairs bile flow and fat digestion
- Disrupts the microbiome via Shikimate pathways
- Kills off beneficial bacteria, causing toxic pathogens to flourish resulting in inflammatory gut disease
- Causes oxalate excess
- Interferes with cytochrome P450 detox enzymes in the liver, leading to accumulation of toxins
- Collagen has a huge amount of glycine in it, disruption leads to osteoarthritis
- Neural tube defects
- Fatty liver disease
- Obesity
- Hypothyroidism
- Iron problems
- Kidney failure
- Insulin resistance
- Diabetes
- Cancer
- Adrenal insufficiency
- PCOS (polycystic ovary syndrome)
- Autism

- Mast cell activation
- Gout
- SIBO (Small Intestinal Bacterial Overgrowth)
- Chelates important minerals: cobalt, iron, manganese and magnesium (they become both deficient and toxic because it takes over and changes the way they are transported
- Interferes with synthesis of aromatic amino acids and methionine
- Glyphosate has a sulfur atom and a methyl group leading to shortages in neurotransmitters and folate
- At just 10 ppt (parts per trillion) it proliferates breast cancer cells in vitro
- 0.1 ppb (parts per billion) alters the gene functions of over 4000 genes in the livers and kidneys of rats causing severe organ damage (this is the level that is permitted in European water supply)
- 10 ppb showed toxic effects on the livers of fish
- 700 ppb is allowable in the water in the US (7000 times more than what is allowable in the water in Europe)
- 11,900 ppb is what was found in genetically modified soybeans
- Autism and dementia are going up in step with glyphosate use

In the US, over 90% of all of the soy, cotton, canola, sugar beets and corn crops are genetically modified while Hawaiian papaya is over 50% genetically modified and yellow squash is now on the list of approved GM crops, as well. This means that any products derived from the above list such as high fructose corn syrup, soy lecithin, cornstarch, maltodextrin and so forth, are also likely to be genetically modified, unless they are specifically labeled as non-GMO or organic. A sampling of non-organic foods containing glyphosate are: Oreo cookies, Goldfish crackers, honey, hummus, Cherrios, wheat based foods, breads, wine and beer. Genetically modified foods have been linked to damage to virtually every organ studied in lab animals. Glyphosate is also found in vaccines, in fact, the MMR-II by Merck was found to contain 2.90ppb, VARIVAX Varicella by Merck contained .41ppb, the ProQuad MMR contained .43ppb, and the Energix-B Hep B vaccine by GSK contained .33ppb.[3]

Dr. Stephanie Seneff's research found that bentonite clay, activated charcoal, sauerkraut juice (probiotic foods) and humid and fulvic acids were able to reduce glyphosate in cows. Since these are all products that humans can also use, it's suspected that the results would be duplicated in humans with elevated glyphosate.

Probiotic foods like sauerkraut, kombucha, kimchi and apple cider vinegar contain acetobacter, one of the few microbes that can metabolize glyphosate! Dandelion and Barberry have been found to be helpful in "fixing illnesses created by glyphosate" and it was suggested by Dr. Seneff that this was due to the supportive nature of these herbs on sulphate transport.

Important nutrients to consider when aiming to detoxify glyphosate are: curcumin, garlic, vitamin C, probiotics, methyl tetrahydrofolate, cobalamin, glutathione, taurine and epsom salt baths.

Glyphosate is a really complex rabbit-hole, but I would encourage you to take the time to learn as much as you can about how this toxin may be partly responsible for whatever health challenges you are attempting to recover, as it really does have a systemic effect on our health.

Also see "Organic and non-GMO foods" under the "Nutrition."

---

1. Dr. Stephanie Seneff Autism One Presentation and slides https://www.youtube.com/watch?time_continue=523&v=YBuXiIF1QEc
2. Slides from Dr. Seneff's Autism One presentation https://www.dropbox.com/s/3dvzaq098b2wvgz/SeneffAutismOne2019.pptx?dl=0
3. A. Samsel and S. Seneff. *Journal of Biological Physics and Chemistry* 2016;16:9-46. A Samsel and S Seneff. *Journal of Biological Physics and Chemistry* 17 (2017) 8-32

HAND SANITIZERS & ANTIBACTERIAL SOAPS

You'll see a variety of these everywhere from public restrooms to doctor's offices, gymnasiums, and even the entrances of department and grocery stores. The intent is a good one, it's an attempt to reduce the spread of germs (bad bugs) on the things we touch the most. Unfortunately, the products being used do more harm than good. One commonly used hand sanitizer is Purell. The Environmental Working Group rated this product, and the ingredients range from a safety index of 1 to 9 on a scale of 1-10! Some of the concerns listed for these ingredients are: developmental and reproductive toxicity, biochemical or cellular changes, cancer, organ system toxicity, allergies, immunotoxicity, irritation of the skin, eyes or lungs, neurotoxicity, ecotoxicity, get the point? Do you really want to put this on your baby's hands, or even on your hands?

Toxicity aside, the other concern with hand sanitizers and antibacterial soaps is that they are not selective about the bacteria they kill and by wiping out the good bacteria on your skin, you are eliminating an important protective barrier designed by your incredibly smart immune system. The beneficial microbes on your skin are the first line of defense in protecting your body from invaders. We want to encourage the survival of the good guys, not wipe them out, we need them! If you wipe the slate clean with the products that kill bacteria, you are only leaving the skin defenseless and vulnerable to other "bad guys" in the environment. Now, that virus or bacteria you picked up by touching the handle to the door at the post office or grocery store is free to multiply and hang around on your defenseless skin, waiting for you to touch your mouth or rub your eye. Next thing you know, you're sick.

It's easy to get caught in the fear-mindset that the product we use to kill off the bad bacteria is saving us from harm, especially when advertising creates this story around why we "need" this product...

when in fact, it's doing just the opposite. Bacteria build up resistance and mutate as a form of survival to man-made chemicals in the environment, and then they pass that genetic code on to future generations of microbes, so that they are also immune to the chemicals. Microbes have been on earth longer than humans, and something tells me they will also outlive humans. They cannot be wiped out by chemicals.

We must fight nature with nature. Nature already has the solutions needed to balance the ecosystem. Our job is to educate ourselves on the natural options available to us.

Although there are many "natural" forms of hand sanitizers available, and I appreciate that they are less toxic, we still must always consider the good bacteria when we choose anything that is intended to kill off bacteria. Not all natural products are selective in only killing the bad bacteria, so in effect, we could be doing the same harm to our protective barrier on the skin, as we would be doing with its chemical counterparts.

My family has chosen to use a probiotic spray as hand sanitizer. Using probiotics instead of products aimed to kill, improves the beneficial bacteria counts on our skin, warding off the bad guys naturally, and without harmful toxic ingredients. I suspect we will see more and more of these hitting the market as their popularity (and our knowledge) grows. We simply use the mist spray on our hands from PureBiotics. I pour some into a little hand sprayer that I keep with me. Another brand that makes a travel sized hand sprayer is Probiotic Power, but their spray has additives that might affect the super sensitive. There is also a brand of probiotic soap and shampoo called Mother Dirt, which is great for cleansing the whole body. You will find links to these websites further on in this resource guide.

The point here is to start thinking more about balancing the harmony of our ecosystem (environmentally and individually), rather than trying to wipe out bacteria that we will encounter day in and day out, all around us. Bacteria lived long before us, they've evolved because of us, and they have proven to have better survival skills than us. We aren't going to eradicate them, so let's learn to live in harmony by balancing out the good with the bad.

HEALING BATHS

Baths have been used for centuries to promote healing and aid in rejuvenation. There is no better way to decompress, destress, supply nutrients and detox in one sitting! Your skin is the largest organ of your body, also known as the third kidney, and bathing offers a unique opportunity for detoxification without putting extra strain on organs. There are many ways baths can be used to promote healing, besides the mere fact that it feels incredibly indulgent and soothing. To amp up the effects of detoxification, try dry brushing before your bath which will stimulate the lymphatic system and increase circulation.

BAKING SODA BATHS

The alkalizing qualities of baking soda make it a great addition to your baths! It is also beneficial for anything affecting the skin, like acne, rashes and yeast infections. Simply add 1/2-1 cup of baking soda to your bath and soak.

CLAY BATHS

There are many forms of clay available, but bentonite clay tends to be the clay of choice for detox baths. Safe and effective for drawing out toxins and stimulating the lymphatic system, clay has been found to pull out heavy metals, pesticides and even radiation. And since clay baths have the ability to pull out toxins through the pores, rather than dumping them into the blood stream, it is a safe way to detox. Adding even just a few tablespoons of bentonite clay to all baths is recommended, if you have chlorine and fluoride in your water, to prevent these chemicals from being absorbed by the skin. Just be careful about letting clay go down your drain which can cause plumbing problems.

EPSOM SALT BATHS

Adding a few cups of epsom salt to your bath promotes drainage and stimulates detoxification. Epsom salt contains a lot of magnesium which is great for aches and pains, but also supports the body's elimination pathways. Because epsom salt is also high in sulfur, those with sulfuration pathway genetic mutations like CBS may have trouble with epsom salt baths though, so if it's more stimulating than relaxing, consider trying a different bath on this list.

HYPERTHERMIA BATHS

"Give me a chance to create a fever and I will cure any disease." -Parmenides

A hyperthermia bath is the act of taking a bath at the warmest temperature tolerated (not scalding!), with the entire body, except for the head, submerged in the water. The intent is to artificially increase body temperature just a few degrees in the way a fever would. Putting a hat on the head improves the hyperthermic effect by reducing the amount of heat released from the head. Since this causes extreme sweating, *it's very important to hydrate sufficiently*, as you would for a sauna. Hyperthermia is used in the treatment of cancer, in fact, there is an entire section about hyperthermia on the National Cancer Institute's website. According to the NCI, *"research has shown that high temperatures can damage and kill cancer cells, usually with minimal injury to normal tissues,"* referring to a 2002 study done in the Netherlands that found that temperatures in the 104-111°F were deadly to cancer cells. Hypothyroidism is known to reduce core body temperature and when overall body temperatures are reduced by even one degree, there is a decline in immune function. Hyperthermia can create a system reset.

A pilot study conducted in Germany and published in the Complementary & Alternative Medicine journal where the participants sat in a hyperthermic bath for approximately 30 minutes each, twice per week for four weeks, concluded that there was significant improvement in depressive symptoms and sleep quality, especially in severely depressed patients.[1]

We know that heat (fevers) kill off infections, so it's no surprise that when we connect the dots between mental illness and pathogenic microbial overgrowth, it makes sense that hyperthermia baths would improve such scenarios. Add in a big dose of probiotics after the body cools down, and you have yourself an awesome (and practically free) therapy. Remember to add a few tablespoons of bentonite clay if your water contains chlorine and/or fluoride to prevent your skin from sucking up those toxins. Hot water can also be drying, so applying a nice oil to the body while the skin is still wet post-bath, is a good idea. Then rest for 15-20 minutes while the body resumes its regular core temperature.

MAGNESIUM CHLORIDE FLAKE BATHS

Magnesium is needed for about 90% of the chemical processes in the body and most people are actually deficient in magnesium. Magnesium baths are a superior way to get your magnesium, over supplemental magnesium, because it is best absorbed through the skin. It is also quite moisturizing, as an added bonus.

MUD BATHS - see "Torf Moor mud baths" in "Nutrition."

SEA SALT BATHS

Sea salt baths are one of the oldest healing baths known to mankind, and one of my personal favorites on this list. Sea salt is an alternative to epsom salt baths if you can't use epsom salts because of aggravation or mutations in the CBS gene. We combine Redmond's sea salt and magnesium chloride flakes for our younger son's bath, since he is homozygous for the CBS gene mutation and doesn't tolerate epsom salt baths. Instead of calming him down, they instigate hyperactivity. Sea salt added to your baths creates a mineral soak that can improve lymph flow by cleaning the lymph nodes, aids in detoxification, boosts the immune system and encourages a healthy exchange of minerals by absorbing them into the interstitial fluid via skin absorption.

A word of caution when it comes to salt baths, be sure you know the toxicity levels of the salt you choose, because the pores are a two-way street. Redmond's sea salt was third party tested by my biological dentist (along with many others) and was confirmed to be on of the least toxic salts of the bunch she had tested. Sadly, Himalayan sea salt, by comparison, had the highest level of arsenic contamination and is often touted as a healthy salt. So know your salt before you soak!

Other things you can add into any bath - Apple cider vinegar, hydrogen peroxide, essential oils, ginger, activated charcoal, witch hazel. Get creative!

I personally mix a few of the above baths together often. One of my favorites is to use sea salt, baking soda, magnesium flakes and essential oils together for a nutritive, aromatic, detox bath. The same principals used above may be applied to foot baths, if full baths are not an option. If you are fighting an illness or have chronic lower body temperature (or cancer) hyperthermia baths combined with a good probiotic (after the body cools down) are a great way to reset the immune system. I love to combine hyperthermia baths with Torf Moor mud baths during the winter months.

Be sure to drink lots of water, before and after your bath. Hydration is necessary for effective detoxification. The warmer the water, the more powerful the detox effect will be.

---

1. J. Naumann, J. Grebe, S. Kaifel, T. Weinert, C. Sadaghiani and R. Huber. *Effects of hyperthermic baths on depression, sleep and heart rate variability in patients with depressive disorder: a randomized clinical pilot trial.* Complementary & Alternative Medicine. 2017; 17: 172. Published online 2017 Mar 28. doi: 10.1186/s12906-017-1676-5

HEAVY METALS

I wish I was referring to the kind of heavy metal my children insist on blaring from the speakers in their rooms, but instead, this subject heading is about the insidious bioaccumulation of metals from our environment. The sources and exposures of heavy metals are countless and growing by the day, many of which we've gotten so accustomed to encountering, that we don't even think twice about their potential for harm.

Your beloved car, for example, it gets you everywhere you need to go, it provides you with a freedom you would never want to be without, but did you know that your car is a host to dozens of chemicals and heavy metals? These toxins become airborne and tend to settle in the dust, so regular cleaning and vacuuming of the interior of your car can reduce a lot of exposure. Opening your windows (especially when you turn on your air conditioning) for a few minutes when you first enter your car, especially if it's sitting in the hot sun, is another technique for reducing toxic exposures normally found in the cab. And also know that while many love diesel fueled vehicles because they are more economical, they do not actually run "cleaner" unless you consider mercury exposure clean.

Heavy metals are not only deleterious to our health because of the biological effects they have on our bodies, but they are also conductors of electromagnetic fields (see more about EMF in "for the home and body" further along in this resource guide). A good number of children on the spectrum have excessive levels of stored heavy metals when tested, my children (and self) included. They are generational, meaning that babies are being born with elevated levels of heavy metals from their parent's and grandparent's exposures.

I don't plan to get into too much detail about the sources of heavy metals, because this list would be endless, but I will plant the seed of awareness with a few tidbits about everyday sources. What you will notice is that we are encountering thousands of sources every single day. Instead of letting this upset you, use this information to fuel your desire to consider a regular means of maintenance detoxification. Our bodies are designed to cleanse themselves, but the onslaught of toxins are just too frequent for our bodies to keep up with. Heavy metals bioaccumulate in tissues and organs, especially when the volume in the blood is too much for the body to eliminate safely. Many of the other headings in this resource guide address options for detoxifying heavy metals, safely. It is VERY important to educate yourself excessively before messing with heavy metal detoxification, because it is possible to redistribute metals.

The more common environmental heavy metals you will encounter are: lead, aluminum, mercury, antimony, arsenic, cadmium, nickel, tin, bismuth, barium, and uranium.

Common sources:

LEAD - old paint such as house paint before 1977, batteries, some solders, some toys, especially antique or imported, glazes on ceramics (look for plates without color or glazes), leaded joints on water pipes, open burning of waste, computers, artificial turf, artificial Christmas trees and lights, curtain weights, jewelry, pewter, pool cue chalk, vinyl, tobacco and second-hand smoke, ceramic studios and industrial smelting and alloying. Deficiency in zinc, calcium or iron may increase the uptake of lead.

ALUMINUM - cosmetics like deodorants and make-up, aerosol formulations of cosmetics, aluminum cans, cookware, aluminum foil which imparts upwards of 400mg of exposure per use in cooking applications, some herbal products, some stainless steel thermos cups, and of course, vaccinations. Silica is capable of detoxifying lead, as well as limiting it's solubility.

MERCURY - amalgam fillings (50% by weight), contact lens solution, hemorrhoid cream, fluorescent (CFL) bulbs, fish (the larger the fish the more concentrated), liquid thermometers, barometers, batteries, fungicides, pesticides and herbicides, coal and petroleum industry emissions, diesel fuel emissions, hospital and municipal incinerators, and some vaccinations still contain mercury. Even if a vaccine is labeled as mercury-free, it may still be used in the production of many vaccinations, then it is removed. This leaves behind trace amounts, and because mercury and aluminum are synergistic, the combination is concerning.

ANTIMONY - tobacco, plastics, battery electrodes, ceramics, pigments, firearms, and it is prevalent in the fireproofing of textiles all throughout your home like curtains, children's pajamas which are not fitted, upholstered furniture, carpeting, pillows, car seats, mattresses, vehicle exhaust etc.

ARSENIC - pesticides, insecticides, herbicides, agricultural soils (which effect rice), chicken feed which contaminates chicken, ground water used for drinking and/or irrigation, sea-living organisms, Himalayan sea salt, preservation of lumber used for outdoor structures like decks, play structures, fence enclosures, and picnic tables built before 2004. If they have a greenish tinge, there is a good chance they were treated with arsenic.

CADMIUM - pigments and paints (including those used on dishes), cookware, batteries (Ni-Cd), plastics, synthetic rubber (found frequently in car interiors), some toys, jewelry, metal coatings, cigarettes and second-hand smoke, dental acrylics, some shellfish, kidney meats, grain cereals and even vegetables, electroplating, mining and smelting activities, photographic and engraving processes. Zinc and vitamin E are protective against cadmium.

NICKEL - bra hooks, cell phones, guitar strings, jean studs, kitchen utensils, musical instruments (keys, mouthpieces), pens, pocket knives, razors, scissors, zippers, belt buckles, chrome and brass fixtures, coins, eye glass frames, yellow and white gold, cigarettes, diesel exhaust, foods, especially cocoa, chocolate, soy products, nuts, and hydrogenated oils, batteries (Ni-Cd), dental materials, electroplating, costume jewelry, pigments for ceramics and glass, and catalyst materials for the petroleum and petrochemical industries.

TIN - dyes, pigments and bleaching agents, biocides used against rodents, fungi, insects and mites, curing agents for rubber and silicone, tin cans, metal alloys, and drinking water piping materials. Tin is commonly elevated in Autistic patients and is often found synergistically with mercury toxicity.

BISMUTH - components of pigments, paints, glazes for ceramics and glass, automatic sprinkler heads, medications, and some cosmetics, like lipstick.

BARIUM - diagnostic testing contrast agents, pigments in paints and decorative glass, insecticides, fireworks, magnets, fluorescent bulbs, welding, glass TV screens and computer monitors, rubber production, some paints, in the water purification process, and there can be very high levels in peanuts.

URANIUM - ground (drinking) water, nuclear fuel, ceramics, colored glass, especially antique, yellow-colored glass.

IONIC FOOT BATH - IONCLEANSE BY AMD

As I mentioned previously under the "chlorella" heading, the IonCleanse was pivotal in our ability to handle detox with chlorella and cilantro. It requires a financial investment, but the testimonials from families with children on the spectrum and with PANDAS/PANS are astounding, making this product well worth it's price tag. They also have a money back guarantee, eliminating the risk of losing your investment if it's not working out for your family. What I found encouraging about a good majority of these testimonials is that even older children had marked improvement, some even using more language!

Two pilot studies were done by the Thinking Moms' Revolution (TMR), a non-profit organization aimed at Autism (and other disabilities) recovery awareness.

During TMR Study #1, the parents of each participating child completed 5 ATECs. A baseline ATEC was completed and submitted prior to the start of the study. Subsequent ATECs were completed and submitted after 30 days, 60 days, 90 days, and 120 days. The average change of the ATEC scores for the 24 participants was a 35% reduction.

Study #2 aimed to test a theory, originally developed by members of the Thinking Moms' Revolution, that increased session times and frequencies with the IonCleanse® by AMD could lead to improved results as measured by the ATEC. This evaluation also introduced a population of older children not included in Study #1.

- *Overall average reduction in ATEC scores was 55% over a 120-day period.*
- *Increased session times and frequencies as laid out in the study design improved results over the previous evaluation.*
- *The greatest average reduction in ATEC scores was in the 13 to 19-year-old age group.*

- *There were no significant differences in males vs females.*
- *100% of study participants showed gains as well as reductions in ATEC scores.*

Study #1 and Study #2 provide strong, statistically significant evidence to support the theory that detoxification with the IonCleanse® by AMD helps children with Autism spectrum disorders. Further evaluations, including double-blind, randomized, placebo- controlled studies, are likely needed to gain acceptance into mainstream Autism treatment programs. Scientists understand that observation can lead to new and improved treatment protocols. While this evaluation, which includes mostly empirical evidence, supports a particular thesis, it is with great hope that other credible research entities will attempt to replicate the studies' findings in controlled, clinical environments. Parties interested in conducting further research should contact AMD directly.[1]

Ionic foot baths effectively change the PH of your body from acidic to alkaline (which has been confirmed via urine PH testing) and the detox continues to alkalize the body up to 48 hours after the treatment, via urination and sweat. It is especially beneficial for people who have gastrointestinal disorders, skin conditions, fungal or yeast infections, and cancer. Detoxification via this route bypasses the GI tract, virtually creating it's own detox channel, another win for methylation challenged folks like us!

Detoxification of this kind dates back 5000 years in the Eastern Indian tradition of Ayurvedic Medicine, where they used concentrated sea salt baths to draw impurities out of the body. Through ionization, where the water is charged with both positive and negative ions (acting similar to the concentrated salt in water), results are much more dramatic in shorter periods of time. The electrolysis combined with added sea salt creates positive and negative ions. The toxins in the feet, which are actually charged particles, are naturally drawn to their opposite charge in the water. Voila, detox, just add water…and salt!! There are other brands, but I can't speak to their safety or efficacy merely because I only have experience with IonCleanse.

Side Note - Foot detoxes are contraindicated for people who have seizures.

---

1. Thinking Mom's Revolution Study - IonCleanse by AMD Part 2, (Dec. 2015) - https:// thinkingmomsrevolution.com/wp-content/uploads/2016/02/TMR-Study-2-Whitepaper-ATEC-Changes-with-the-IonCleanse-by-AMD.pdf

LYME DISEASE

There is something referred to as Lyme-Induced Autism (LIA) and should be part of the exploratory phase of any Autism recovery. Likewise, on the other end of the spectrum (pun intended) Lyme Disease has been indicated in some Alzheimer's misdiagnoses and should be considered whenever autoimmunity and neurological symptoms have been triggered as a potential contributor. PANS can be caused by or be in part related to Lyme Disease, as well. Since studies, along with growing evidence, suggest there is an ability for Lyme disease to be transmitted via bodily fluids (the Lyme bacteria has been found in saliva, urine and breastmilk) it would be wise to recognize Lyme disease as an important box to tick (pun intended) for any weaknesses identified in the immune system.[1] Lyme disease is tricky to pin down, again because of its incredibly intelligent and morphological nature.

A negative Lyme test does not necessarily mean a person doesn't have Lyme disease. It is for this reason that I would recommend processing your testing through IgeneX Inc., as they are the most thorough and effective lab which has specialized in detecting Lyme disease and its many co-infections for over 25 years. I also highly recommend looking into Dr. Klinghardt's work on recovery from Lyme disease. He is pioneering successful treatment with the most up to date research on how to heal from this devastating illness. He has recently discovered a unique correlation between Lyme Disease and retroviruses. You can find more on his website at KlinghardtAcademy.com.

---

1. R.B. Stricker & M.J. Middelveen (2015) *Sexual transmission of Lyme disease: challenging the tickborne disease paradigm*, Expert Review of Anti-infective Therapy, 13:11, 1303-1306, DOI: 10.1586/14787210.2015.1081056

MOLD

Anyone and *everyone* with health issues involving the immune system should absolutely consider the possibility of mold in their environment, not just their home, but any environment frequented on a regular basis. About 25% of the population has a specific genetic mutation in the HLA-DR genes, predisposing them to sickness from water damaged buildings. Their body doesn't recognize mold toxins as foreign, causing these toxins to accumulate rather than being excreted. HLA-DR genes tell your body to make antibodies to fight toxins. Without them, your body could not remove these toxins. For these people, the antigens remain in the body causing global inflammation leading to multi-system symptoms known as CIRS (Chronic Inflammatory Response Syndrome).

Unfortunately, it is very common to have mold growing indoors, especially in newer style homes, because of the more recent building practices used.

Mold can begin to grow on a porous substrate within 24-48 hours of water exposure, if it is not properly ventilated and dried out. Mold is microscopic until it grows out of control, so just because you don't see it, doesn't mean it isn't there. Also, having no active and obvious leaks, doesn't mean you are out of the woods either, because hidden leaks can be brewing inside walls without visibility. We had three of them, which probably began when our home was built based on the location and the extent of the damage. There were very tiny, dripping leaks behind the walls, and it wasn't until the problem escalated under unique circumstances that we saw visible evidence of the leaks on the interior of the home. Once we dug into them, it was clear that these leaks had been going on for years, unbeknownst to us.

The damage was so extensive that there was over a foot of wood rot in the subfloor from the exterior wall extending inward, but it was not even visible from the unfinished ceiling in the basement. In this particular incident, when I pulled back insulation that was covering the hidden wood rot along the outside wall framing, there was a huge mushroom growing on the wood! This is probably the exception to the rule, but I can't tell you how many stories I've heard from people about water coming into their homes and their idea of fixing it is to caulk, paint and move on. This is a sure fire way to ensure the growth of mold within the wall cavity, especially in homes with insulation and sheetrock. Once mold spores are in the air, they are free to enter the heating and air conditioning system where they get blown all over the house. The spores attach themselves to surfaces where they just sit and wait for the right conditions to begin growing enough to become visible. Since mold is microscopic, it takes quite a bit of growth for it to become visible to the naked eye.

A question I hear a lot is, "if there are molds outside, isn't it unreasonable to expect our homes to be mold-free?" Yes and no. So yes, there is mold outside and yes it does enter our homes on our bodies and feet, but there is a significant difference between outdoor mold and mold from a water damaged building. Certain spores are more common in a water damaged building and some of these strains, like Stachybotrys (aka - black mold) are much more dangerous when they multiple uncontrolled in an indoor environment than the strains we are exposed to outside. It's true that an outdoor mold can become elevated in a house for various reasons, but the more concerning strains and quantities come from water damaged buildings.

Our son's worst PANDAS/PANS flare was triggered by exposure to mold, both in our home and at his school concurrently. Remediation at home and pulling him from school, in combination with using homeopathy, camel milk and soil based organisms to help his body clear the toxins brought him back to baseline. However, we still had a lot of work to do to detox him further.

Remember that mold can be anywhere, not just in your home, but also in schools, libraries, therapy buildings, doctor's offices, work places, even cars, RVs and boats, etc. They must all be considered if the person spends any time in the environment regularly.

The standard method of testing in the industry is air captured, which is only a small representation of what is going on in your air, in that particular room, during only that particular moment in time. There are many heavier molds that don't spend much time in the air and various conditions can effect testing. For example, Stachybotrys and Chaetomium are heavier molds and spend only about 90 seconds airborne. Considering these are also two of the most lethal water damaged building strains, you will want to consider testing that captures settled spores as well. The more ideal representation of the mold index of a home is captured by an ERMI test. It uses vacuum or fabric to swipe for sample collection from dust that has settled on surfaces in the home, and the results are much more accurate (assuming you captured the best samples possible), because they test for the DNA of the mold strains in the dust samples.

When it comes to remediation, it is very important to be educated *before* you touch anything! Do your research. You are better off letting mold be than tearing open a wall to see what is going on without proper containment. Once you disturb mold, the spores are like dandelion seeds blowing in the wind, they will release into the air and attach to surfaces around the building or home. Once these spores get into your porous furnishings, they are considered contaminated. Only non-porous surfaces can be cleaned and even then, the types of mold in the environment make a big difference in how or what you decide to clean.

If you are dealing with Stachybotrys or Chaetomium, these are sticky molds and very hard to clean from just about any surface. So, if you are going to consider remediation and you even remotely think there could be mold involved, hire a good company to contain the area even before any extensive exploration is undertaken, ideally.

They should construct 6-mil plastic walls and run a negative air machine inside the containment with ventilation to the exterior in order to prevent excessive cross contamination within the home. When the remediation process is complete, they need to use a HEPA vacuum to clean the entire inside of the containment before breaking it all down and removing it safely. I highly recommend going the extra mile if the area you plan to work on has ever had a leak (even small) or if you think the area might contain mold.

You can't undo the exposure once you start messing around with it.

It's also very important to understand how mold responds to threats, because you can make matters worse, if you decide to "kill" mold rather than removing the moldy porous substrate. Attempting to kill mold forces it to release potent mycotoxins, in an attempt to kill its threat, which are neurotoxic and are usually more problematic than the spores themselves. These mycotoxins can't be cleaned off easily and typically have a half-life of over 90 years, which means in 90+ years, only *half* of the mycotoxins will decompose.

I repeat, *if you don't have the proper safeguards in place, don't mess with mold!* I've mentioned other products in this resource guide for dealing with environmental mold, before, during and after treatment. Once remediation is complete, it may be necessary to detox the body from the effects of mold, which can also grow inside the body. Elevated mycotoxins being stored in the body require effective detoxification. Doctors Richie Shoemaker and Dietrich Klinghardt have paved the way for mold toxicity recovery. If you are a victim of mold toxicity, begin your research with them. There are also many great social media groups connecting people who have been through various stages of recovery. Please also see my section on "Air Purifiers" under "Toxins" in the resource guide of this book for ways of reducing mold in the environment as you work out your plan for remediation, as well as controlling cross contamination post-remediation.

See my website AskHealthyJess.com for more information and products I recommend for mold.

PLASTICS

Plastic is all around us, so it is hard to completely avoid, but do what you can to replace plastic with cadmium-free glass where possible. Plastic around food is the biggest concern to our immediate health, but the consequences of our gross overuse of plastics are showing up in landfills and garbage dumps, our water supply and our oceans where they will cause long-term damage to our ecosystem, as well as infiltrating our food supply. The atmosphere we live in is recycled so we must consider every environmentally stable toxin to be a long term threat to our planet.

Rolf Halden, Associate Professor at the School of Sustainable Engineering at Arizona State University, and assistant director of Environmental Biotechnology at the Biodesign Institute once said,

> *"Today, there's a complete mismatch between the useful lifespan of the products we consume and their persistence in the environment."*

Testing is confirming suspicions that our environmental exposures have cascaded to the point of effecting just about everyone. Plastics are present in our blood and urine in measurable amounts, even in newborn cord blood. Plastics are hormone-mimicking endocrine disruptors with links to numerous health conditions including developmental problems, early onset of puberty, immune system suppression, liver dysfunction and precancerous growths. To make matters worse, the health liabilities are magnified in children whose organs and immune systems are still developing. At minimum, avoid plastic baby bottles, teethers, cups, kitchenware and whatever you do, never heat food in plastic containers, which increases leaching![1]

---

1. J.L. Carwile, H.T. Luu, L.S. Bassett, D.A. Driscoll, C. Yuan, J.Y. Chaang, X Ye, A.M. Calafat and K.B. Michels. *Polycarbonate Bottle Use and Urinaary Bisephenol A Concentrations*, Environ Health Perspect. 2009 Sep; 117(9): 13681372. Published

online 2009 May 12. doi: 10.1289/ehp.0900604, PMCID: PMC2737011, PMID: 19750099

RIFE MACHINE

Rife machines are named after Royal Raymond Rife. Rife's claim to fame came from two specific inventions (although he had many others). One was a powerful microscope capable of magnification claiming to be as high as 31,000 times. The second invention was an electromagnetic therapy device consisting of a light transmitter feeding a plasma tube (Tesla tube) that killed pathogenic microorganisms at specific frequencies according to their own electromagnetic "signature."

In 1932, Rife succeeded in isolating a "filter-passing" microorganism (later referred to as the BX virus) that was a cause of cancer. He opened a clinic where he cured all (16 of 16) cancer cases within three months by targeting the microorganisms with his light frequency machine. Sympathetic resonance states that if two similar objects are near each other and one of them is vibrating, the other will begin to vibrate and will entrain to the first, some examples are: tuning forks, grandfather clocks, guitar strings, even women living together start menstruating at the same time.

Essentially, the rife machine mimics the quantum frequency of a microbe, causing it to vibrate, resulting in its destruction. Once a microbe has been killed by the rife machine, the immune system recognizes the antigens on the dead pathogens as an unwanted life form and creates T-cells and B-cells to kill all the other pathogens with those same antigens anywhere else in the body. It's been estimated that the rife machine kills about 50% of your pathogens and the immune system kills the other 50%. While the T-cells are reabsorbed soon after the pathogen is gone from the body, the B-cells live for 60 years and will go into action if the same type of pathogen ever tries to invade your body again.

Anthony Holland discovered that cancer, including leukemia, uterine and breast cancer, and even MRSA (the antibiotic resistant strain of bacteria) is easily destroyed at frequencies between 100,000 Hz and 300,000 Hz. In targeted, lab tested experiments, he was able to show actual cancer cells and MRSA being destroyed by resonant frequencies. Prior to their destruction, they grow blisters, swell, explode, disconnect and break apart. A simple search in YouTube of *"shattering cancer with resonant frequencies Anthony Holland"* will result in microscopic videos from a cancer lab.

Rife machines have come a long way since the 1920's and can now target numerous toxins, as well as microorganisms, encouraging detoxification from the body. The key to doing this successfully without a severe Herxheimer effect (healing crisis), is to run multiple frequencies together, including frequencies that target healing in the body while supporting healthy and effective detoxification. This is not a quick fix and it ideally should be paired with the use of binders and supplements that support the organs responsible for the detoxification process.

Under the guise of quantum entanglement, the Spooky2 rife machine takes rifing to the next level by allowing treatment from a distance. Quantum entanglement uses the premise that when DNA is separated from its host, anything you do to the separated DNA will have an equal effect on the host. This enables treatment as you go about your business, rather than having to be connected to or in close proximity to the device. Lyme and cancer patients rave about the results they've had with the Spooky2.

I personally had an interesting experience with the powerful combination of our Spooky2 rife machine and homeopathy. This experiment was completely unintentional. I had been running biofeedback scans weekly on myself. I used the remote treatment on the machine to treat myself with these results for the entire following week. Then I would do it all over again, the next week. New results, new treatment.

Two months into using it, I was identifying a new homeopathic remedy for myself and after narrowing my selection down to three remedies, I decided to blind muscle test them to decide on the final remedy. The remedy that was selected was the cancer miasm nosode, Carcinosin, which has the ability to address the susceptibility to cancer (and symptoms associated). It doesn't require a person to HAVE cancer to need this remedy, just expressed susceptibility symptoms that suggested that I was expressing the miasm (as mentioned earlier in the book).

What I found interesting was that every biofeedback scan I conducted on myself up to this point resulted in multiple cancer hits. In fact, the scan I had done prior to using the cancer remedy resulted in eleven cancer frequencies coming up for treatment. Again, just like with homeopathy, this doesn't mean a person HAS cancer, but it does indicate a possible susceptibility, so I immediately wondered how my next scan would look after using the remedy for an entire week.

The first biofeedback scan after taking my cancer miasm nosode remedy resulted in only ONE cancer frequency. In all of my scans, this had never happened before. It was very clear to me that not only did the remedy effectively begin to clear my susceptibility to cancer, but the rife machine was incredibly in tune with this shift!! What an incredible confirmation that these modalities do indeed work and using them together can be powerful.

WATER

There is no denying that hydration is essential for life, but what we don't think about often is how clean that water is. Township water adds chlorine and fluoride (in many cities) and the contaminants are too many to list, while well water has organic matter to contend with. In either case, it's a good idea to safely filter and structure your drinking and cooking water, at minimum. If you can also filter your bathing/shower water, that would increase the healthy water your body is absorbing. Studies have confirmed that healthy cells are surrounded by structured water, while unhealthy cells are surrounded by chaotic water molecules, aka unstructured water.

Water in nature is structured naturally by its surroundings by running over rocks and soil. This is definitely an area that warrants your research. We chose to use a structured water filtration system. There are many systems on the market so it can be confusing, but I would recommend taking the time to become well educated in your options because some can actually cause more harm than good. We chose AquaLiv, because it structures the water and the filtration is efficient, yet doesn't eliminate minerals from the water, like reverse osmosis does (although they do also offer a reverse osmosis system). Eliminating minerals from your water is a dangerous practice, because drinking water devoid of minerals will actually leach minerals from your body! This will slowly deteriorate your health.

Structured water increases the pH of water and counteracts toxins, as well as providing your body with water the way nature intended it to be. I tested our structured water with a digital pH meter and found it to be about 8 to 8.5. A pH of 7 is considered neutral, while higher (7.1-14) is alkaline and lower (0-6.9) is acidic. An overly acidic body is prone to illness while an alkaline body is protective. It is completely normal (and necessary) for the pH of stomach acid to be slightly acidic, while the blood is slightly alkaline. Food effects the pH of your urine and excreting acids in your urine is one of the main ways your body regulates blood pH.[1]

It is also important to find a filter that specifically reduces fluoride, because most do not. If you don't want to install an under sink filter, ProPure and Berkey have great water tank options. You can get travel sized tanks, but even the full size tanks pack up nicely for transportation. They would be great to take to hotels where you can't be sure about your water quality. These tanks are designed to handle filtering stream water, so they are very effective. We take our own water everywhere we go, whenever possible. We fill Life Factory glass bottles with water for on the go all the time.

---

1. "The Alkaline Diet: An Evidence-Based Review," https://www.healthline.com/nutrition/the-alkaline-diet-myth#osteoporosis

WRINKLE-RESISTANT FABRIC

Do you ever think about all the wrinkle-free shirts in your closet or those easy-care sheets you just bought? What makes them wrinkle-free or easy-care? They certainly aren't grown that way. (wink) Although we may be attracted to the ease of caring for garments and sheets labeled as wrinkle-resistant, the risks outweigh the benefits here. N-methylol Acrylamide and DMDHEU resin are commonly used in the treatment of wrinkle resistant fabrics. These chemicals produce free formaldehyde, which has been identified as a carcinogen, and can also cause detrimental dermatological effects. Remember that the skin is an absorbent organ. Do you want your loved ones engulfed in formaldehyde all day and night?

ZEOLITE

I wish I knew about clinoptilolite zeolite before I had my children! This is one of the gentlest ways to detoxify the body. Natural zeolite is a volcanic mineral that can cleanse a wide range of toxins from your body. Zeolites have the ability to sort molecules based on size, as well as molecular charge. The honeycomb structure has a negative charge within each of its chambers, which attracts positively charged toxins like heavy metals, mycotoxins, histamines and pesticides, among others.

Since your body cannot store zeolite, it will bind with toxins as it harmlessly passes through your body and out...with the toxin. Don't let the door hit you on the way out! In order for it to be effective at adsorbing toxins, it is very important to be sure you are either using a cleansed natural zeolite or a well-made synthetic zeolite, so that it doesn't already have bound toxins in its honeycomb matrix.

Evidence suggests that other benefits to zeolite is that it alkalizes the body, strengthens the immune system by increasing T-cell activity and the number of macrophages in the body, supports a healthy gut by increasing the integrity of the intestinal wall and it has antimicrobial, antiviral and anti-fungal properties! Some are concerned about zeolite when they discover that it contains an alumina molecule, but fear not, these molecules are tightly bound into the honeycomb structure where they will stay. More technically according to Coseva, the manufacturer of Advanced TRS which is a synthetic form of clinoptilolite nano-Zeolite,

"Some of the quadri-charged silicon is replaced by triply- charged aluminum, giving rise to a deficiency of positive charge. The charge is balanced by the presence of singly-and doubly- charged atoms, such as sodium (Na+), potassium (K+), calcium (Ca2+), and magnesium (Mg2+), elsewhere in the structure. For manufactured clinoptilolite, atoms or cations (charged metal atoms) aluminum and silicon are

known as structural atoms, because with oxygen they make up the rigid framework of the structure. This is why the form of aluminum in zeolites is completely inert and does not react or release in the body in any way. Sodium and potassium are known as exchangeable ions, because they can be replaced (exchanged) more or less easily with other cations in aqueous solution, without affecting the aluminosilicate framework. This phenomenon is known as ion exchange, or more commonly cation exchange. The exchange process involves replacing one singly-charged exchangeable atom in the zeolite by one singly- charged atom in a solution or replacing two singly-charged exchangeable atoms in the zeolite by one doubly-charged atom in a solution."

The only risk of breaking these molecules apart *may* be if you take hydrochloric acid (HCI) alongside of the zeolite. Research suggests that supplemental HCI can break apart zeolite molecules, so I would recommend avoiding this combination! Natural stomach acid, however, hasn't shown to have this same influence on the zeolite matrix, according to studies. There are numerous studies on the impressive benefits of clinoptilolite zeolite. Go ahead and do some digging, because you will want this stuff in your medicine cabinet, better yet…on your counter!

$\mathcal{N}$UTRITION

JUNK IN, junk out. Have you ever heard that saying? Well, it's true. We get out what we put in. Nutrition is paramount to a healthy body. Our bodies run on nutrition just like a car runs on fuel, so redefining what is nutritional to your body is a requirement you can't overlook when coming up with a healing regimen. For children nutrition is even more essential due to their developing brains and body. The food we eat is used to form the cells and tissue in our bodies. I know you want to provide your child(ren) with the best possible foundation for growth and development.

EVEN IF YOU are doing great things to heal your body, if you are feeding it junk or things that cause disruption in the ecosystem, you might not experience deep and permanent healing. In homeopathy, dietary issues are considered maintaining causes, meaning no matter how accurate the match to your remedy is, you might experience a block to healing, because your vitality isn't strong enough to overcome the continuous deficiencies of your diet.

CAMEL MILK

When I tell people we drink camel milk, I often get a puzzled look, a pause, then the question, "Did you say Chamomile?"...and then when I slow it down and say it once again they always seem to follow up with, "But if you react to milk, how do you drink camel milk?" Yes, camel milk is milk, BUT it's very different from cow's and goat's milk. It has medicinal properties that have been healing people at record speeds for centuries, and now they have found it can also help people with diabetes, allergies, cancer, Autism, mast cell disorders, histamine intolerance and more. Studies are confirming these findings. There is still a small amount of lactose in camel milk, but the lactose is even different, and much easier to digest than cow's milk lactose.

In raw camel milk, the enzymes remain in tact, allowing the person to digest the lactose more effectively. The problem with lactose often stems from drinking pasteurized milk, which is denatured and lacks the enzymes necessary to digest the lactose. We cease to create the enzymes necessary to break down dairy products shortly after infancy, so it is actually quite normal to not tolerate milk as we age past infancy.

The proteins in camel milk are the decisive healing components, because camel milk contains no beta-lactoglobulin and it has a completely different beta-casein – the two components in cow's milk that are responsible for allergies to milk. Camel milk contains a number of immunoglobulins that are comparable with human immunoglobulin, although they are referred to as nanoglobulins, because of their size. The camel nanoglobulins mimic the human immune system. They are minuscule in size by comparison, but look like ours. Their size allows them to cross through cells so when you drink the milk, you are filling your blood (and intestines) with these healing nanoglobulins. This is like having an IVIG (intravenous immunoglobulin) treatment with camel milk!

Camel milk is also rich in vitamin C (five times as much as cow's), calcium and iron (ten times as much as cow's milk). It has a good amount of calcium, healthy levels and ratio of omega 3 and 6 and it contains more lactase for those who have trouble digesting lactose. The healing properties are numerous, from the amino acid profile to the enzymes and minerals!

There are four components that have come to light in studies with camel milk and it's these components that enable it to rehabilitate the immune system:

- The Lysozyme enzyme which strengthens the immune system and fights pathogenic microbes
- Oligosaccharides, which aid in cell recognition and binding, serve as probiotics and support gut healing
- Secretory IgA which (along with the Lysozymes) protects against pathogen, allowing the repopulation of the good guys and
- Lactoferrin (an iron sugar that is an immune system modulator), which is antimicrobial and supports nourishment and healing of the gut over time.

An added benefit is that camel milk is rich in antioxidants and the ASD population is historically deficient in antioxidants. As you navigate the camel milk options that are now available throughout the world, you will want to understand the topic of raw versus pasteurized more thoroughly. Clearly there are benefits with all raw milks, versus pasteurized, but even so, the complexity of balance with heating the milk enough to reduce the pathogen load while retaining immune components must be considered. There is often a trade off, depending on the procedures used to process any raw product. The question of pasteurized versus powdered is a tricky one too, because either can be processed in favorable and unfavorable ways. Any high heat product is discouraged, with raw being the ideal product, but it is also recognized that there are many factors at play, with each person's individual needs driving their decisions. Even an imperfect camel milk will offer more nutrition than other substitute milks like rice milk which contain added ingredients and sugars.

The four components of camel milk must be considered when choosing a raw or pasteurized product. Heat sensitive components that are damaged during heat processing are Secretory IgA and Lactoferrin. Components that are minimally or unaffected by heat are Lysozyme enzymes and Oligosaccharides. There are freeze dried camel milk options for those who don't have access to fresh or frozen raw milk. The benefits of this form of processing is that no heat is used and many of the nutrients are able to be kept in tact. In the case of diabetes, camel milk offers a rich source of absorbable insulin, which was never thought to have existed before these findings. This is why insulin is injected rather than taken orally. Scientific evidence is confirming that camel milk reduces fasting sugar and reduces post granular glucose and HBA1C, which enables type 1 and 2 diabetics to cut down on medication.

At the time when we began using camel milk medicinally, Gavin had been diagnosed as failure to thrive. He was small from birth and although he maintained a bell curve in growth, he just remained very small in size. He had been at a standstill remaining at 10% for weight and 2.2% for height. In the first two days of starting the camel milk, he gained 3 pounds!! I had weighed him just days before starting it (because I weighed him almost daily back then, lol) and then two days later his weight went from 27-30 pounds overnight! I kept waiting for this extra weight drop thinking it would be temporary, but even when the kids were off the milk for a long weekend, the weight remained!

I had read about how it increases bone density and in studies it caused the same kind of immediate weight gain in another child, from the absorbable calcium it provides. He continued to gain weight, although at a much slower pace than this initial spurt. Within a month, his growth chart percentages went from 10% to 46% and his height went from 2.2% to 7%. His weight quadrupled and his height tripled! It was astonishing! Grayson grew too, although at a much slower and consistent pace. In that same month, he went from 10% in height to 13% and from 23% in weight to 33%.

Beyond this, the behavioral changes were equally as astonishing, we saw huge cognitive changes in both boys, they became more talkative, more inquisitive, much more aware and engaged in their environments and their humor bloomed almost overnight. My blog contains a lot more detail about our experiences with camel milk. The experience wasn't perfection from the start, because there was a period known as a healing crisis, where things temporarily got worse before they got better. There was a mix of improvements with the die off responses, but the intensity of the immediate improvements had us wanting more. We used camel milk medicinally (a pint a day for each) for about 9 months, then we backed off and began using it much like you would use milk, as a food. Now we enjoy making smoothies, ice cream, candy, camel milk lattes, cereal, and anything else you would do with a milk product. It's nice to have something other than alternative substitute "milks" which aren't milks at all, and generally contain a lot of fillers and unhealthy additives.

I'm sure you are wondering, where can I get this liquid gold? Back when we began using it for our boys, I found only 3 farms in the USA, two of them right in our state. We made an event out of driving to the farmers to pick up our milk. Since then, the access has changed considerably and you can now access camel milk quite easily. Since there was so little awareness of camel milk when we were using it, my friend and I created a Facebook group called *Healing with Camel Milk* which had a handful of members for a while, but then as the awareness grew, so did the group. Within seven years, we had grown to over 12,000 members worldwide, and the list of 3 farmers I originally knew of in the USA, grew to over 12 and a total of 24+ resellers worldwide (and is still growing)!

Note - Always ask your supplier for proof of testing for pathogens, if you choose raw milk.

CELL SALTS

There are 12 homeopathic bioplasma cell salts and according to Dr. Schuessler, these 12 minerals are crucial to the health of the body. They include forms of calcium, iron, potassium, magnesium, sodium, and silica that work at the cellular level; hence, the name "cell" salts. Deficiency in of any of these minerals will cause an imbalance in the body.

Homeopathic cell salts offer a safe way to rebalance the minerals that are out of balance. We have taken the 12 in one Bioplasma product, but using them individually has significant benefits too. A great book that guides us in the use of them individually, as needed is called, "Natural Healing with Cell Salts" by Skye Weintraub, ND. You can look up the ailment and find a list of cell salts that are beneficial for that ailment. Then you can read about each of those cell salts to see if you can identify which would be related to the cause of the ailment. When trying to rebalance minerals, it's a good idea to use the appropriate cell salt(s) daily for at least a few months. In some cases, supplementation with the coordinating mineral can supply the body with the mineral while the cell salt works on proper absorption of that mineral. Cell salts are adaptogenic, meaning they can help balance minerals that are either too high or low.

CHLORELLA

In addition to chlorella's uncanny ability to assist in detoxification, it is also one of the most balanced nutrients available on the market, and rivals synthetic multivitamins, without a doubt. It is the only known plant source of B-12 that we can digest and it contains more B-12 than a T-bone steak. Chlorella is one of the richest foods in protein, beta carotene, nucleic acids (RNA & DNA) and it contains more chlorophyll than any other food and since it assimilates instantly due to the algae's predigestion of it's protein and beneficial fats, it is more likely to be utilized effectively by the body. Due to its acid polysaccharides, it is also an immune booster. It sure appears to live up to being a superfood! Because we also take cilantro tincture for detoxification, which can mobilize more metals than it can eliminate, this is another reason to have chlorella on board. We take chlorella thirty minutes prior to cilantro tincture and then follow-up with a good binder an hour or two later, to be sure everything that was mobilized exits the body.

See more about chlorella in "Toxins."

**CAUTION - do *not* disrupt heavy metals in the body using products like chlorella, cilantro or any other "chelator" if you currently have metal/amalgam fillings in your mouth. Not all metal-containing fillings are silver. White fillings can contain high amounts of metal as well. They would be evident in an x-ray by glowing white. Resin fillings don't glow white in an x-ray.

DIETARY CONSIDERATIONS

Dietary interventions hold a lot of consideration and should be examined in *every* scenario where health is suffering, in my opinion. There are so many dietary insults that could potentially be masking as illness, or worse, triggering degeneration, that it should be the first consideration out of the gate. You can't repair the inflammation, if there are constant inflammatory assaults going on multiple times a day.

Leaky gut, also known as intestinal permeability, is caused by lifestyle choices and when we are exposed to toxins on a day-to-day basis, we don't give our body a chance to heal, because the resulting daily exposures create chronic inflammation. Research has demonstrated a link between intestinal permeability and exposure to: alcohol, pharmaceuticals, especially antibiotics, trans-fats, GMO foods, plasticizers, food dyes, high-sugar foods, chlorinated water, pesticides and herbicides such as Glyphosate. A study conducted by scientists from China's Shandong University found that just four weeks of supplementation with B. longum, L. acidophilus, and S. thermopiles reduced intestinal permeability.[1] Supporting the microbiome is essential to good health, which starts in the gut.

What we eat becomes our fuel and it literally creates our cells and tissue. Let's look at a few dietary interventions that have been successful for chronic illness. Again, this isn't meant to be all-inclusive, but rather some breadcrumb droppings designed to get you inspired and researching more. There is nothing more empowering than becoming more educated.

GFCFSF - I consider gluten-free, casein-free (dairy) and soy-free to be absolutely essential and it should categorically be THE starting point when attempting to recover from any autoimmune disease or neurological ailment. The reason for all three is because their protein shapes are so similar that the body confuses them for one another so when a person has a sensitivity to one, the body is also most likely sensitive to the others (even if you haven't figured that out on your own yet). Gluten, dairy and soy may not be the only foods causing problems, but they are the biggest offenders more often than not. In addition to causing hyperactivity, spaciness, sensory dysfunction, cognitive decline, joint pain, chronic headaches, eczema and changes in personality, food sensitivities are also known to cause chronic fatigue, migraines, back pain, fibromyalgia, psoriasis, acne, diarrhea and constipation.

Please be aware that "gluten-free" according to the food industry does NOT mean *free* of gluten. The food industry has a predetermined threshold of gluten considered to be "gluten-free" and for some, that threshold may be too much. If you prefer to eat foods that are truly free of gluten, you will want to know exactly what you are eating. A food that is prepackaged or labeled as "gluten-free," is not necessarily free of gluten and for some people, even trace amounts can cause inflammation throughout the body and/or an opiate effect. Gluten remains in the body for 6-9 months and in that time frame, if we continue to expose ourselves to industry standard "gluten-free" foods, imagine the accumulative effect.

There may never be TRUE healing if we don't fully eliminate certain gluten-containing products from our diets. We must be our own food detectives. If you are trying to eliminate gluten and you REALLY want to give gluten-free eating a shot (to see if it resolves health problems) I think it's imperative that this detail be taken into consideration. The only true gluten-free diet is created by cooking your food, in your kitchen, with your own fresh ingredients. A great place to find more detailed and step-by-step guidance on this is on the website TACAnow.org. TACA can guide you with all the tools needed to take the step towards allergy-friendly cooking and eating healthy.

LOW OXALATE DIET (LOD) - The kids and I have problems with the build up of oxalates, which can eventually lead to kidney stones, if not managed sufficiently. Unaddressed, it can also lead to kidney failure, requiring dialysis, so it's not something to take lightly. This is unfortunately also quite common in the Autism population, partly due to bacterial imbalance. A study published in the Journal of Endourology confirms the effects specific antibiotics have on the Oxalobacter formigenes bacteria which is solely responsible for the degradation of dietary oxalates. In recent testing, it was confirmed that I am lacking in O. formigenes colonies. These are not currently a strain that can be replenished via commercial probiotics, because they are anaerobic, which means they don't survive in an oxygen-rich environment, aka - out of the body. Thankfully though, there are a few companies working on such products, so it appears be an option we may see in the future. It is without a doubt, one of the more important reasons why we must preserve the good bacteria we have, encouraging their propagation.

Killing off bacteria thoughtlessly leads to a diminishing O. formigenes population. The deposition sites of oxalate crystals are commonly the: eyes, kidneys, thyroid, heart, joints, urinary organs and locations of previous injury, but they can really deposit anywhere.

Oxalate crystals look like little miniature fishing hooks, can you imagine what that does to the surrounding tissue? If you have joint or muscle pains, aching all over, back or neck pain, frozen shoulder, problems with pain in your eyes (feels like grit or sand), burning, red or crusty eyes, floaters in the eyes, painful or unnaturally warm urination, cloudy urine, frequent urination, chronic lower back pain, kidney pain, bladder pain, gallbladder pain, "sandy" or gritty stool, burning stool, light colored stool, black specs or white crystals in stool, IBD, chronic UTIs, air hunger, heart palpitations, peripheral neuropathy, burning tongue/mouth, sinus issues, odd sensations like fullness in the ears, vertigo and dizziness, tinnitus, fluctuations in hearing, frequent rashes, ravenous hunger, chronic candida overgrowth, carpal tunnel, CFS, arthritis or fibromyalgia, you really should experiment with the low oxalate diet to see if it brings relief.

THE FAILSAFE DIET - Stands for Free of Additives and Low in Salicylates, Amines and Flavor Enhancers. Like oxalates, other food chemicals can be naturally occurring compounds found in foods. Through a significant elimination trial, we discovered that our younger son doesn't tolerate most of the foods addressed in the Fail-safe diet which fall under the categories of: Salicylates, Amines, Glutamates, and additives like food coloring and preservatives. Sensitivities to food chemicals are dose-related rather than immune-mediated like allergies.

The symptoms can involve the central nervous system, the endocrine system, the gastrointestinal tract, the genitourinary system, the head, eyes, ears, nose and throat, the heart, the immune system, memory, musculoskeletal system, the skin, sleep, speech and the vascular and pulmonary systems. Just one infraction and the reaction in our younger son was almost instantaneous and resulted in intolerable behaviors like: aggression, impulsivity, hyperactivity, obstinance, defiance, excessive anger, lack of focus and even violence in some cases. Additional accumulative exposures caused him to progress into other symptoms like headaches, fatigue, hypo-glycemia, and he became unreasonable and unmotivated. His anger and obstinance undermined everything he did when he was inflamed from these foods.

We have been able to soften the blow using Ness Amylase enzymes when he's had minor, singular infractions, but overall, the best course of action is avoidance. This is a common diet that is used successfully with children who have been diagnosed with ADHD, ADD, Asperger's syndrome, PANDAS/PANS, dyslexia, OCD, ODD, and learning difficulties. For our younger son, this was THE biggest piece of his ability to remain functional. If your child falls into any of the above categories, an elimination diet is warranted. It has been life-changing for Gavin, no, let me rephrase that, it is abso-lutely essential for Gavin! I know there is a lot of talk about raw diets being the next best thing for improved health, but for kids like this, a raw diet would severely increase many of the food chemicals that they react severely to.

OTHER DIETS - There are many other specific diets that address gut healing. We haven't used these other diets, just the ones that have made sense for our family, but you will likely find plenty of information if you research the diets that have produced healing for others. Some of the more common diets are: GAPS, SCD, low phenol, The Body Ecology Diet, etc. I tend to steer clear of any diets that aim to starve out yeast. Candida albicans (a yeast) is a normal resident of our microbiome and it serves a very important purpose.

Starving Candida is akin to using pharmaceuticals, in that it aims to eliminate symptoms rather than going after the reason the overgrowth occurred in the first place. I agree with not feeding unhealthy foods that directly feed fungus/yeast like refined sugar, but I completely disagree with removing a food like fruit, with the sole purpose of trying to starve out Candida. First of all, fruit is the food with the highest vibration and contains natural sugars that our body actually needs. When we starve a yeast like Candida, it actually becomes more virulent and grows tentacles in an attempt to protect it's species (and remember, we actually want it to be a part of our microbiome in normal proportion). In this virulent state, it becomes much harder to control. The tentacles will literally be driven through the intestinal wall, creating holes and ultimately results in intestinal permeability. So yes, yeast overgrowth can be the cause of intestinal permeability, but we must be careful not to mistake this "cause" as the root cause.

Why is the Candida overgrowth there in the first place? Eating high-sugar diets is certainly a recipe for disaster and can increase Candida colonies, but if you've reduced refined sugars and simple carbs and there is still a problem, you must consider the possibility that there are other toxins involved, as the role of candida in the body is to sequester these toxins in an attempt to protect you from them. Reduce your incoming toxins and provide gentle detoxification opportunities and you will see the yeast overgrowth normalize. This was the one tried and true method that worked for us. In our case, the Low Oxalate Diet actually eliminated the boys' chronic systemic yeast overgrowth. I personally required more than just the LOD.

So how do you get started with dietary intervention?

This all seems so overwhelming when you are just beginning, doesn't it? This is something you must approach one day at a time, don't think too far into the future. Address only what you can today. When you take it one step at a time, it isn't as daunting as it appears from the overall perspective. So let's break it down:

Breathe first

Big deep breaths!! It CAN be done and it WILL become habit. Your new shopping list and recipes will be second-nature before long, I promise. We all had to start somewhere.

Research

Go online and hit all the websites that detail recipes and alternative foods. Read, read, read!

Lists

Make lists of all the foods the child CAN have and there really are still a lot of foods available. Make lists of the foods the child cannot have, including and even more importantly the list of *hidden foods/ingredients* to avoid and keep those in a bag that is with you always, for the sake of shopping. You will need to refer back to these on many occasions. *Make a copy of them to give to close relatives and care givers who interact with your child.*

Recipes

Find recipes online, from friends, and in books that address special diets (you will probably need to learn how to substitute certain ingredients), make grocery lists from there initially, eventually you will just be replacing those items as you run out. It becomes second-nature to shop for these foods. In the early days I found it helpful to keep a running list, as I ran out of a food, I would write it down. Now, I have a generic list that I typed up and I just check off the foods I need as I run out.

Talk with your child through it all

I am amazed at how well a three-year-old can really comprehend what this is all about. We told Grayson he couldn't eat foods from the "red list" (the color of the reactive foods on his IgG food panel repot) and how they effect him. I believe that by feeling better on the good foods, he also gets to experience the natural consequences of eating the foods he can and can't have. When he has an infraction, he feels the effect more than we do. His outward behaviors are just a sign of what is going on inside.

Journal

Keep a daily journal that not only details foods and supplements, but keep track of improved and difficult behaviors, you will start noticing connections to certain things that can further be eliminated. This is also important when choosing to challenge a food. The other great thing about a journal is that you will be able to look back at the progress you are making with the diet. It is easy to forget the difficult behaviors until you are faced with them again. Something that helped me was to use color coding highlighters with one color for improved/good behaviors, one for difficult behaviors and another for the first three times foods were introduced during the diet, so I could watch for patterns with a quick glance of the pages. When you have umpteen pages to sift through, this will save your sanity!

Connect

Find a local or internet-based group you can share with and learn from. Facebook offers us endless reaches around the globe, instantly. There is nothing better than having a resource like this. When a question pops up, you can gain knowledge from those who are directly effected by the very same issues you are faced with. It's a two-way road, you will learn from others who are more experienced than you, and eventually you will help others who are newer at it than you. I find this method of learning to be priceless and rewarding in many ways.

And last - make the switch - go shopping

We went cold turkey, but for some, a gradual approach works best. Be aware that changing the diet drastically can create some symptoms of detox. Either way, just go for it and don't look back. When you offer your child a new food, it must become the ONLY option. The good thing about children is that they tend to have narrow food interests, so once you find a food to replace a favorite, maintaining the diet is actually pretty easy!

Imagine that? Comfort and ease come with repetition. We initially experienced resistance with two favorites - milk and bread. So basically, we didn't offer any!

A note about preparing meals - Whether you realize it or not, while you are cooking, you are infusing the water and food you are preparing, with your current vibration, therefore, it's imperative to take note of the mood you are in while preparing meals for your family. If you are stressed about new dietary changes, take some time to recenter yourself before cooking. Eating out also means that you are subject to the mood of the chef and others handling your food. One more reason to eat healthy organic foods made in the home. We also like to add written affirmations to our bottled water jugs, fermented food containers and even on little notes to carry in our pockets or put into pillow cases at night.

Enzymes

At some point, consider researching and adding digestive enzymes to the diet. Generally, food intolerance is related to the lack of an enzyme needed to digest the food(s) which causes a leaky gut, resulting in antibody production. Adding enzymes for a good two months while on the diet may allow you to return some food(s) to the diet slowly, and possibly even permanently. There is more information than you could ask for on EnzymeStuff.com.

Go to my website AskHealthyJess.com for links and more guidance on dietary interventions.

---

1. Zeng J, Li YQ, Zuo XL, Zhen YB, Yang J, Liu CH, *Clinical trial: effect of active lactic acid bacteria on mucosal barrier function in patients with diarrhoea-predominant irritable bowel syndrome*, Aliment Pharmacol Ther. 2008 Oct 15;28(8):994-1002. doi: 10.1111/j.1365-2036.2008.03818.x. Epub 2008 Jul 30

IODINE AND IT'S CO-NUTRIENTS

The most thorough explanation I have found regarding the many reasons for needing iodine are in a book by Dr. Brownstein, "Iodine, Why you need it, Why you can't live without it." In addition to the details in this book, we are also facing a world where radioactive iodine has been released into the atmosphere via Chernobyl and Fukushima nuclear fallouts. Testing has confirmed the presence of radioactive material in drinking water, grass, cow's milk, mushrooms, fish, and so on. Without the proper saturation of nutritive iodine in our bodies, our uptake of the radioactive form of iodine is significant. Proper iodine saturation in our bodies prevents the uptake of the radioactive form. To add insult to injury, chlorine and fluoride as well as brominated products will displace iodine from our bodies, increasing our deficiency. Improper iodine saturation leads to microbial imbalances, infertility, thyroid disorders and many forms of cancer. It is VERY important however to know how to properly supplement with iodine so please don't just run out and buy iodine to take without researching what co-nutrients are necessary for proper balance.

JUICING

We aren't die-hard juicers, because of the oxalate build-up potential of many fruits and vegetables, but we do like to have an occasional fresh juice, because of the high impact nutrient delivery it offers. It's like a shot of nutrients that go straight to the blood stream! Be sure to look for masticating juicers since it preserves the nutrients and enzymes, where as the centrifuge heats and destroys the enzymes and nutrients which is counterproductive to the reason you are choosing to juice. They have come down quite a bit in price since the originals were developed and are very affordable health gadgets to have in the house.

If you happen to notice new symptoms after beginning a juicing routine, be sure to compare those symptoms to oxalate dumping symptoms which can include: joint or muscle pains, aching all over, back or neck pain, frozen shoulder, problems with pain in your eyes (feels like grit or sand), burning, red or crusty eyes, floaters in the eyes, painful or unnaturally warm urination, cloudy urine, frequent urination, chronic lower back pain, kidney pain, bladder pain, gall-bladder pain, "sandy" or gritty stool, burning stool, light colored stool, black specs or white crystals in stool, IBD, chronic UTIs, air hunger, heart palpitations, peripheral neuropathy, burning tongue/mouth, sinus issues, odd sensations like fullness in the ears, vertigo and dizziness, tinnitus, fluctuations in hearing, frequent rashes, ravenous hunger, chronic candida overgrowth, or carpal tunnel. An increase in any of the above symptoms might suggest you are not degrading oxalates and therefore are accumulating them, resulting in a pattern of dumping oxalates. If this looks familiar to you, see the Low Oxalate Diet section of "Dietary Considerations" in "Nutrition."

ORGANIC NON-GMO FOOD

I doubt this really needs any explanation, just do your best to eat organic and non-GMO as much as possible. This goes for meats also! Look for organic, grass-fed and free range meats. If your budget is tight, you can find natural meats that eliminate the use of antibiotics and hormones at minimum and follow the top 10 lists for the most crucial organic produce to consider. It goes without saying, what you put in directly effects what you get out...junk in, junk out.

The health risks associated with eating genetically modified foods are mounting as the crops are growing. GMO crops are laden with an insecticide known as Roundup, of which the main ingredient is glyphosate. Glyphosate has just been declared by the World Health Organization (WHO) as a possible carcinogen.

According to Jeffrey Smith, Institute for Responsible Technology Founder, creator of the documentary "Genetic Roulette" and participant of the docu-series, The Truth About Cancer, Roundup can promote cancer in many ways. Glyphosate is essentially an antibiotic, killing off beneficial bacteria, resulting in an overgrowth of bad bacteria, promoting inflammation. This overgrowth has been linked to cancers like colorectal, stomach and gallbladder cancers, as well as lymphoma. The overgrowth of bad bacteria results in an endotoxin known as Zonulin, which promotes leaky gut as well as leaky brain. Undigested proteins in the brain result in autoimmune disease. When glyphosate was originally patented in 1964, it was meant to be a chelator of trace minerals, magnesium especially, which has been shown to be another probable cause of cancer.

Our beneficial bacteria use something known as the Shikimate-acid pathway to produce essential nutrients like folate and aromatic amino acids that our bodies can't make. These amino acids are precursors to all kinds of biologically active molecules in our body.

Glyphosate blocks the Shkikimate pathway. Promoters of glyphosate debate that there are no ill effects to humans, because we don't have a Shikimate pathway, but the residents of our microbiome do and they are essential to our lives.

One of the most troubling concerns associated with ingesting glyphosate is that it is a synthetic amino acid and glycine analog which can become incorporated into proteins in place of glycine. What does this mean? It means that glyphosate is pretending to be glycine. There is a code for glycine and because glyphosate looks just like glycine, it gets picked up. It fits right into the glycine socket perfectly. Glyphosate then gets in the way, disrupting enzyme function, therefore the proper enzymatic reactions won't happen, in other words, these functions become non-operative. Glycine is normally used in DNA and RNA transcription, protein and enzyme synthesis and collagen formation. Dr. Stephanie Seneff of MIT said,

> *"An amino acid analog of glycine clobbers all life. Glyphosate is the only glycine analog that exists."*

An overview of the potential harmful effects glyphosate is responsible for, according to research conducted by Dr. Stephanie Seneff of MIT:[12]

- It is a synthetic glycine analog, allowing it to get into proteins
- DNA/RNA dysregulation which ultimately disrupts mitochondrial function and ATP production
- Interferes with the sulfation pathway which is essential for excreting toxins like aluminum, mercury and xenobiotics
- Disruption of sulfate synthesis and transport also impairs bile flow and fat digestion
- Disrupts the microbiome via Shikimate pathways

- Kills off beneficial bacteria, causing toxic pathogens to flourish resulting in inflammatory gut disease
- Causes oxalate excess
- Interferes with cytochrome P450 detox enzymes in the liver, leading to accumulation of toxins
- Collagen has a huge amount of glycine in it, disruption leads to osteoarthritis
- Neural tube defects
- Fatty liver disease
- Obesity
- Hypothyroidism
- Iron problems
- Kidney failure
- Insulin resistance
- Diabetes
- Cancer
- Adrenal insufficiency
- PCOS (polycystic ovary syndrome)
- Autism
- Mast cell activation
- Gout
- SIBO (Small Intestinal Bacterial Overgrowth)
- Chelates important minerals: cobalt, iron, manganese and magnesium (they become both deficient and toxic because it takes over and changes the way they are transported
- Interferes with synthesis of aromatic amino acids and methionine
- Glyphosate has a sulfur atom and a methyl group leading to shortages in neurotransmitters and folate
- At just 10 ppt (parts per trillion) it proliferates breast cancer cells in vitro
- 0.1 ppb (parts per billion) alters the gene functions of over 4000 genes in the livers and kidneys of rats causing severe organ damage (this is the level that is permitted in European water supply)

- 10 ppb showed toxic effects on the livers of fish
- 700 ppb is allowable in the water in the US (7000 times more than what is allowable in the water in Europe)
- 11,900 ppb is what was found in genetically modified soybeans
- Autism and dementia are going up in step with glyphosate use

In the US, over 90% of all of the soy, cotton, canola, sugar beets and corn crops are genetically modified while Hawaiian papaya is over 50% genetically modified and yellow squash is now on the list of approved GM crops, as well. This means that any products derived from the above list such as high fructose corn syrup, soy lecithin, cornstarch, maltodextrin and so forth, are also likely to be genetically modified, unless they are specifically labeled as non-GMO or organic. A sampling of non-organic foods containing glyphosate are: Oreo cookies, Goldfish crackers, honey, hummus, Cherrios, wheat based foods, breads, wine and beer. Genetically modified foods have been linked to damage to virtually every organ studied in lab animals. Glyphosate is also found in vaccines, in fact, the MMR-II by Merck was found to contain 2.90 ppb, VARIVAX Varicella by Merck contained .41 ppb, the ProQuad MMR contained .43 ppb, and the Energix-B Hep B vaccine by GSK contained .33 ppb.[3]

Get more informed and get involved with the non-GMO revolution at the Institute for Responsible Technology at responsibletechnology.org.

---

1. Dr. Stephanie Seneff Autism One Presentation and slides https://www.youtube.com/watch?time_continue=523&v=YBuXiIF1QEc
2. Slides from Dr. Seneff's Autism One presentation https://www.dropbox.com/s/3dvzaq098b2wvgz/SeneffAutismOne2019.pptx?dl=0
3. A. Samsel and S. Seneff. *Journal of Biological Physics and Chemistry* 2016;16:9-46. A Samsel and S Seneff. *Journal of Biological Physics and Chemistry* 17 (2017) 8-32

ROTATION DIET

Due to the nature of our restricted diets, it was also essential to rotate the foods our boys could have. If we had just given them the same handful of foods day after day, they would have also become sensitive to these foods, because of the repeated exposures. The rule of thumb here is to avoid a food for three days before eating it again. With leaky gut syndrome, it can become a vicious cycle, because if you expose the body to the same food over and over, the process which caused the problem in the first place continues and the killer T-cells which have already become cytotoxic via activation from an antigen will target these new foods. Cytotoxic cells typically target bacteria, viruses, tumor cells, or other cells of the body, but in the case of leaky gut, they are triggered by repeating food offenders. These reactions may also be involved in some delayed hypersensitivity reactions, such as celiac disease, in which there is a reaction to the gliadin fraction of grains and wheat gluten, as well as potentially causing damage to the mucosal lining of the gut or even contribute to protein wasting conditions, like celiac disease, ulcerative colitis, and Crohn's disease. So, what has worked well for us is to feed the same foods for two consecutive days, then take a three day break from them before going back to them. To make life easier, we created a schedule to follow which keeps us on track. The kids know it by heart and automatically know which snacks they can have accordingly. It has become just another part of our routines. As mentioned earlier in the book, according to testing, the rotation diet allowed ten food sensitivities to drop off of Grayson's IgG food panel, and Gavin has never developed more than four food sensitivities because he has eaten this way his entire life.

TORF MOOR MUD BATH

Who doesn't love playing in the mud? I know, a bath doesn't sound like nutrition, does it? When you are sitting in a hot bath, your pores open up and amazingly, you are offered the opportunity to introduce nutrition through the skin! Torf organic mud (also known as therapeutic peat moss) baths from Austria, Hungary and Czechoslovakia contain more than 1,000 herbs, plants, grasses and flowers that have decomposed over a period over thousands of years, turning it into a nutritious soup of vitamins, minerals, plant-based hormones and other phytonutrients. Research has shown that the mud can help to improve circulation, stimulate the immune system, break down fat cells, soothe aching muscles, reduce swelling in joints and it's anti-bacterial. Some claim that drinking it can calm and heal the gut. Others even believe it can help infertility. It is a strong detoxifier, due to chelation abilities that enable it to bind to heavy metal isotopes. My kids love taking mud baths, it's complete irony, a bath with mud in it!

$\mathcal{L}$IFESTYLE

Your lifestyle (the way in which you choose to live your life) determines your daily flow and defines how you overcome obstacles. It is the basis for all of our decisions. Our choices and habits, conscious or subconscious, have the power to create our reality, therefore alterations in lifestyle have lasting effects, positively and/or negatively. Upbringing, culture, religion, interests and opinions play into the lifestyle habits we create. It begins at brith, evolving as we age, and reflects our attitude, way of life, values and world views. A healthy or unhealthy lifestyle is often disseminated through generations. You can see that our lifestyle really contains the roots of who we are, therefore, living consciously and mindfully has an impact on every aspect of our lives. One might argue that our lifestyle dictates our personality.

In the list below, I will share the various tools in our toolbox which were responsible for developing a healthier lifestyle. Just like the other sections of this resource guide, the topics are arranged alphabetically, not according to importance. Importance is subjective and individual.

AMYGDALA RETRAINING

I've spoken about the importance of changing old thought patterns and how that was a vital part of our recovery. Changing thought patterns is the conscious act of creating new neurological feedback loops, which can also be formally called amygdala retraining.

Amygdala retraining relies on neuro-plasticity to rewire neurological conditioning. If you can imagine yourself in a situation with a predictable outcome, like anxiety triggered by a diagnosis or eating a particular food that causes a predictable reaction, the two events always seem to correlate, don't they? This is in fact what PTSD is at the core, it's the pairing of an event with a a predictable outcome that has the propensity to repeat itself.

Typically there is an initial traumatic event that sets the stage for the pattern, but sometimes the trauma is developed over time with the repetition of two events, reinforcing the neural pathways involved. You might remember when I mentioned earlier in the book about how a little girl eating her ice cream cone, who is attacked and bitten by an aggressive dog, might develop an allergy to dairy from the traumatic event. How does this happen? When two neural synapses fire together, especially when the event is emotional, they create a deep groove in the brain, like a road, also known as a neural pathway. Once this road is paved, it provides a path for easier travel going forward, in other words, it's possible for this paired pathway to become activated when only one of the two events is triggered in the brain, because now the two synapses fire together. It's critical to know also that the more a pathway is used, the deeper the groove becomes.

In demonstration, we can see neurological conditioning played out during a well-known study called, "Pavlov's Dogs." In this study, dogs were first exposed to the ringing of a bell, to demonstrate that the bell-ringing had no effect on their salivation (of course it didn't, why would it, right?). The dogs were then exposed to food, which innately causes salivation. The next step in the study was to combine presenting the dogs with food while ringing the bell, at the same time. This was repeated so that when the bell was rung (without food) the dog's salivation was triggered by the bell-ringing alone. Here we have a prime example of neurological conditioning. For these dogs ringing a bell created salivation, because the two synapses fired together repeatedly, creating a new neural pathway. Anything we repeat, becomes engrained in our neurology in this way. The good news is that neural plasticity is ongoing, and we can retrain our brains with intentional events to replace the old and harmful pathways.

There are formal amygdala retraining programs that can provide you with the intentional focus needed for a more successful outcome. They require one hour of your day for six consecutive months, but these hours can be broken down into fifteen minute chunks throughout the day. While I didn't use a program like this during our recovery phase, I did inadvertently reproduce amygdala retraining in our environment, as needed, using positive, heart-opening thoughts to replace negative, repetitive thoughts. It certainly took longer than 6 months, but it was effective and it came natural when I recognized the patterns. In my opinion, it would be hard to achieve full compliance in a child with one of the amygdala retraining programs, but creativity can go a long way and by using it for yourself, you can mitigate where a lot of these patterns might have begun in the first place.

A combination of modeling the program for your child and using key take away activities during acute flare ups would be a great start to creating a customized program for your child. I plan to consider a formal program to address the food sensitivities (and our negative loops associated with them) that still remain in our family. We have already begun the process by priming our kids with the simple task of replacing negative thoughts with healing thoughts while eating, and placing little reminder notes around the kitchen. I hope this will become second nature for all of us. The takeaway from a program like this is a life long mind-set associated with the power of the mind to recreate the reality we desire. Also see the topic "Mindfulness."

CRYSTALS

My interest in crystals actually developed through Grayson. He has been attracted to crystals since he could notice and grab them. At the age of five, he stopped his little league football game to dig a large piece of quartz out of the dirt below his resting position while in formation. He handed it to his coach to give it to us for him. Even earlier, he would find them in the most unusual places, as if he had radar for them, in the base of planters, in gardening displays, at restaurants and malls. He has been buying them with his own money ever since he could acquire his own money, which says a lot because he didn't often have much to begin with. His fascination grew, pointing me in the direction of discovering the importance of crystals in his life, and mine. They are so much more than just pretty rocks.

Crystals each carry a unique quality of high vibration, which has the ability to entrain your body or parts of your body, to match the crystal. They are powerful absorbers and transmitters of energy, therefore, they also require regular cleansing, although a few are self-cleaning. Crystals form from a variety of minerals creating an orderly, repeating atomic lattice which is unique to it's species, also lending to its color and external structure. The internal structures can be identified under a microscope and it is how geologists identify each crystal.

Certain crystals have the ability to absorb negativity and electromagnetic smog and in return, they put out pure, clean energy. If you find that computers have a negative effect on you or your child, place a fluorite cluster or a piece of lepidolite beside it, which will result in harmony with your computer rather than resistance. Crystals have been used for healing and balance for a millennia. They work through resonance and vibration, and can even be useful for acute conditions, especially when used as a gem essence.

Many modern day uses for crystals go unnoticed, like quartz which is used in watches and as part of the memory chip in computers, and piezoelectric crystals are used to produce sound waves in ultrasound machines. A tightly focused beam of ultrasound can cauterize wounds deep within the body and blast tumors apart without the need for invasive procedures. The applications for crystals span the gamut as wide as the selections of crystals are varied. You can wear them, toss them into a pocket or a bag, put them in the soil of your plants (unless Grayson sees them there), keep them on a desk, in your car, around your kitchen where food is prepared, you can structure water with them, take them as gem essences, meditate with them, put them on an end table or underneath the bed for improved sleep, and so on.

A few of my favorite ways to use the healing properties of crystals, besides just having them around me all the time, focuses on their benefits in the kitchen. I like to place a few around the jars of ferments while they culture and tinctures while they are steeping. I also like to infuse and structure my drinking water with them. In fact, you can buy a travel mug that has interchangeable crystal bases for structuring your to-go water. Since water holds memory, it will take on the structure of the crystals that are either placed just outside of the glass or right into the water itself. It is important to educate yourself on the safety of crystal varieties for this purpose *before putting anything into your water*, because there are some crystals which contain toxic minerals and metals. These would make better homeopathic remedies, if the stone resonates with you, because there are no toxic crude doses in the remedies. Quartz and Amethyst are great for this purpose, but don't limit yourself, explore what additional crystals can do for your particular needs.

ENERGY HEALING

There are many styles and methods of energy healing available, especially since it can often be done long distance, so you virtually have the world of options at your fingertips. Energy Healing is a complimentary modality and can be combined with any other modalities of choice.

Choosing an energy healer is an intimate decision and must come from your intuition, but when you find the right healer for your family, it can be magical.

Also see "Hands-on Healing Modalities."

FAMILY MISSION STATEMENT

Part of our home schooling experience was to create a family mission together, then to memorize it and live by it. We recited it every day and we talked about how real life events fit into our mission. We even made a board game for the family from the basis of our mission as a hands-on way to help the children comprehend how to apply it to our lives, and they love playing it.

Having a family mission is also an inspiring tool for establishing and monitoring a family code of ethics with positive spin and can become an active teaching tool. It can be used to help make big decisions, by making sure your decisions are in line with the objectives of your mission. It can be used to help regain focus and realignment with things that matter most to your family. We all have a mission in life, even if we don't exactly call it that. When used appropriately, a family mission can shape the feeling in the home.

Stephen and Sean Covey offer great advice about writing family missions in their book, "The Leader in Me." They do a nice job of inspiring thoughtful missions by suggesting exploring what your family is all about, and to do that you can ask the following questions at a family meeting:

- What is the purpose of our family?
- What kind of family do we want to become?
- What are our family's highest-priority goals?
- What are our unique talents, gifts, and abilities?
- When are we the happiest?
- What do we want our home to look like, feel like, and sound like?
- What kind of home do you want to invite friends to?
- What makes you want to come home? What would make you want to come home even more?

- How can I/we as parents be more open to your influences?

They go on to encourage a few more helpful tips that include the following:

- Write it as though you intend to live it. Be realistic.
- Consider all four basic needs: physical, social-emotional, mental, and spiritual - thinking about the whole child, the whole family.
- Keep in mind the various ages in the home so that the language and concepts are meaningful to all. I would add here that in our families, with children on the spectrum, we must also consider their comprehension level and communication abilities.[1]

According to Nicholeen Peck of "A House United,"

"A family mission starts with a family who has a vision of what they want to become and take the time to plan for that vision."

Our mission:
We the Galligani family will encourage and foster the change we want to see, both in our home and beyond.

We are dedicated to creating a loving, peaceful and compassionate environment, full of enriching educational opportunities daily.

We lift each other up, provide loving, respectful support for one another, and we extend our outreach to all of mankind with courteous and thoughtful attitudes.

By following the guidance of our own heart and soul, we will graciously and happily fulfill our life's mission together.

---

1. Sean R. Covery, Sean Covey, Muriel Summers, David K. Hatch, *The Leader in Me*, Simon and Schuster Paperbacks (2008)

FREE-PLAY TIME

…and lots of it. Studies are mounting, suggesting that children need more free time to play unstructured. Research from Germany has found that adults who recall have a lot of free time during their childhoods more often experience higher levels of social success as adults. Schools that are increasing recess are seeing a reduction in ADHD and if you research schools from some of the most respected countries, they don't structure the school day for children until they are in high school, because they believe children learn best through play. Free time as kids has also been linked with higher self-esteem. So, please don't over-schedule your child(ren)'s lives, and offer a lot of time for creative play.

HANDS-ON HEALING MODALITIES

There are many hands-on healing choices available: chiropractic care, spinal network analysis, cranial sacral and cranial structural therapy, myofacial release, osteopathic treatments, Reiki, QiGong, massage, acupressure, acupuncture, EFT (Emotional Freedom Techniques), etc.

Choose your practitioners wisely, because you don't want your child taking on any negative energy from the practitioner. In addition to using a few of the above modalities, we chose to become attuned to Reiki, meaning we took the classes to be trained in Reiki which involves an attunement at the close of the classes. Reiki is a great way to treat not only others, but yourself, making it another fabulous tool to add to your self-help toolbox!

Many of the above modalities offer physical and energetic healing in one. Some practitioners are more intuitive then others, trust your gut when it comes to working with practitioners of this kind.

HOMESCHOOLING

If there is one thing that I can definitively say has contributed to the speed of healing in our home, it's homeschooling. I know it isn't available to all families because of the financial drawbacks associated with having one of the parents home full-time, but let's face it, most of our kids learn differently and just don't fit into the public school model. Homeschooling doesn't have to occur during regular business or school hours though, so even in a dual-income family, creative solutions are possible.

Removing our boys from the school system enhanced healing by significantly reducing their exposure to chemicals, foods, microbes and the energy of others who effect our little empaths.It also empowered them to follow their own passions rather than being reminded daily that they must conform in order to be accepted. Homeschooling assists in relationship building at home while enabling our children to find their true interests and build on them without restriction.

We follow a combination of the Thomas Jefferson Education Model and the Charlotte Mason method which encourages a love of learning primarily through reading and exploration. Besides family reading, we also encourage activities and exploration into topics the kids are interested in. Think about your education for a moment, which things have you retained from those early days? I'm going to guess it was either something you loved (and probably still do) or something that you enjoyed the process of learning about, or maybe it was because of the personality of the teacher you had. A good teacher makes learning fun and memorable. Otherwise, you have probably forgotten a good percentage of what you were forcibly taught. When we are interested in what we are experiencing, it is naturally retained and utilized.

Hands-on is the most effective way for children to learn, without a doubt, and at home most learning is hands on. This one-on-one approach allows for much less time to be spent on academics and more time to be spent on personal interests, which also have the ability to expand on the child's knowledge by leaps and bounds. I read an article that broke down the average school day so that the actual learning time could be extracted from the hours kids spend in school. It was about one and a half hours on average!

Homeschooling is focused one-on-one learning and can result in incredible progress without requiring the pressures of replicating the school environment at home. Studies have repeatedly proven that children learn an incredible amount about the world around them through creative play.

JOURNAL YOUR JOURNEY

Journalling is a great way to release unsettling emotions and to dig into the deep crevices of your spirit, as well as documenting your journey for future reference. This can come in handy when you are feeling deflated. When I began to retrace our past events for the purpose of writing this book, I was quickly reminded of how far we have come.

Journalling can come in the form of day to day occurrences or you can journal very specific components of your path like dietary changes being made or supplements added to your routine, etc. By keeping track of changes being made to your routine, you are offered the benefit of a higher level review of the effects your changes have shaped.

I have found it helpful to use color coded highlighters so I could glance back through my notes and see patterns emerging with the highlighter hierarchy.

KINDNESS

For everyone, yes EVERYONE! Your neighbors, teachers, grocery baggers, your boss, even your estranged friend, parent or sibling, everyone! Be kind to unkind people, they need it the most. Harboring hard feelings doesn't only hurt the other person, it hurts you. Anytime you are engulfed in the flames of a negative thought about another person, the frequency of that low vibration thought is being applied to your body at that very moment. Remember, your body doesn't know the difference between real and imagined events. And on the flip- side, kindness benefits you, as well as the other person. This is two-fold actually. You benefit from the initial frequency generated by the action or thought, but then when the other person benefits from your kindness, their reciprocated kind thought sends you more high vibrations and may continue to do so, as this person replays the event or shares it with others.

Anytime a person thinks about you, or you about another, an invisible cord is developed between the two of you, this cord connects you to the vibration of the thought much like a radio station tunes into the frequency being sent to it. You can't see it, but it's there, traveling through the air. So, make a habit of thinking and doing kind things. Random acts of kindness are a wonderful way to lift the spirits of everyone you. Your little gift of kindness might be just what that person needed and could elevate them for the entire rest of the day. I have been consciously doing this for so many years that now that it has become subconscious habit. I can only see the good in just about everything (there are still exceptions, I am human, after all) and it adds vibrant color to my day, it makes me high, quite literally. There is no better high than kindness and love, spread it around and it will come back to you two-fold!

LISTEN THOUGHTFULLY

Your children are probably more in tune with their own bodies than you are. Let them have a voice. You may be surprised by their opinions and advice. Take time to listen to them. Put down the phone, close the computer and look into their eyes. Quality time is fleeting with busy schedules always looming. Take advantage of the opportunity for fully engaging conversation, especially when they initiate it. Before long, they will be grown up and won't need (or want) your advice as often.

MEDITATION

I have probably said enough about meditation already, so I will just reiterate the importance of taking time for you to sit in silence, whether it's 5, 10, 15 or 30 minutes. Whatever you can squeeze out of the day will be enough, so as Nike says, just do it!

If you missed it, go back to Part I, "Meditation does what?" To learn more about the benefits of meditation.

MINDFULNESS

Being mindful is the act of staying present, without criticism. It means you are fully attending whatever you are doing, on purpose. When we are present, we are fully engaged in the experience. When we veer from the present, our mind takes flight. If I am doing the dishes mindfully, it means I am engaged in the process, I am fully focused on the dish I am currently washing, every nook and cranny receiving my attention. I feel the warmth of the water on my hands, I notice little nuances I wouldn't notice if my attention was fleeting. I might also be thinking about how grateful I am to have a reason to wash these dishes (and I take advantage of sharing these thoughts with the children when they are around). I am experiencing the moment 100%. If I zone off into thinking about something else, I've lost connection with the task at hand, I am only half engaged, maybe less. We are more effective and grateful when we are mindful, it represents a conscious mind-set. We can be mindful in all of our actions.

I have used the "MindUp!" books to offer my children mindfulness experiences that will stay with them forever. When we move about the day in mindfulness, there is no room for anxiety or fear. We are filled with the fullness of every moment's purpose. Over time, mindfulness becomes habit forming and has been known to bring about long-term changes in mood, happiness and wellbeing.

If you struggle with remaining present because of overwhelming unhappy conditioning, there are ways to retrain your habits. We all carry around some baggage which can come from our past in the way of repetitive negative thought patterns. A way to create presence and break free from the pain of a particular situation comes from Eckhart Tolle's "A New Earth" and will help with reframing the experience that comes with the thoughts.

First, focus your attention on the feeling associated with the situation that triggers you. Recognize how you feel and know that there is nothing you can do *at this moment* about this feeling. Now, instead of wanting this moment to be different from the way it is (which only adds more pain to the pain that is already there), ask yourself if it is possible for you to completely accept that this is what you feel right now. If you still find yourself unable to accept the feeling, recognize that it is the unhappiness speaking for you. Notice that your unhappiness is about being unhappy, it's just another layer of unhappiness. If you don't mind being unhappy, what happens to the unhappiness?[1]

Repeat this new thought pattern whenever you feel the resurgence of painful thought patterns surfacing. Allowing yourself the grace and power of no longer resisting what is will give you the power to control your thoughts. The dimension of presence will begin to transcend your personal past. Staying present allows us to stay focused on what we need today, on loving and embracing today, without attaching to images of the future which may never transpire, or the past which is gone. These thoughts only cause us pain in the here and now. When we are focused on the past or the future, we aren't available to experience today and today is all there really is! The past and future are only thoughts.

Live today mindfully!

---

1. Eckhart Tolle, *A New Earth Awakening to Your Life's Purpose*, Penguin Group (2006)

MUSIC

Music has always deeply moved me, all the way back to childhood, but even more so as I have aged. Music reaches deep into my soul and pulls out my pain, releasing old stored painful vibrations with each note. Meditation combined with music is like a transformation catalyst for me, encouraging a more eventful and meaningful experience every time. Yoga coupled with music turns a physical exercise into therapy of the mind, body and soul.

Children can have this same experience. Experiment with background music during arts and crafts. I encourage buying children instruments from a very early age. Our boys began playing guitar very young. It wasn't structured for a long time, but when they decided to take it seriously, they began learning songs on their own. We built on their knowledge by putting them in formal lessons when they were ready. They also both play piano now, as well.

Put it on and turn it up! A dance party always has a way of turning the tides when someone is feeling down.

SELF-EDUCATION

Self-education fueled by empowerment rather than worry!

Knowledge is power…as long as we don't use that power to fault ourselves when we can't fulfill every whim we have. I have always found the old adage that "knowledge is power" to be true. It is not only empowering to broaden your foundation of information about subjects that interest you, but it can broaden your horizon, as well.

Follow your your intuitive compass rather than allowing fear to drive your research. Fear- driven research can breed more fear. That isn't to say you shouldn't educate yourself about something you are fearful about, by all means, empower yourself by learning more on the subject, but I would suggest staying away from looking for the drama in the situation. Find solutions, not problems.

I have always been soothed by informing myself, by researching solutions to my problems. Sometimes just knowing there is a solution, or many, is enough to calm my frayed nerves. My entire journey through recovery has been fueled by my need for information, but I've been very careful to use the research I find to encourage beneficial change rather than letting it push me deeper into depression. As an action-oriented person, my research has been the force behind our healing.

SELF-TALK

Self-talk is the inner-dialogue we create with ourselves in our minds, it's that part of our communication that is referred to as the subconscious. It's very important to speak mindfully to ourselves. This internal dialog creates our beliefs about ourselves, and our beliefs about ourselves creates the platform for our actions.

If you find yourself feeling discouraged, you can consciously change your negative thought patterns.

Here are a few positive phrases that will increase your confidence enabling you too move forward from a difficult moment where you feel stuck:

- This is tough, but so am I
- I may not be able to control this situation, but I am in charge of how I respond
- I haven't figured this out...yet
- This challenge is here to teach me something (this is a personal favorite that I use frequently)
- All I need to do is take it one moment at a time. Breath and do the next right thing

SLEEP

This may seem obvious, but I am including it because it is easy to overlook when bad habits have set in, and optimal sleep is paramount to good health, moods and for a well functioning immune system. In children, sleep is responsible for a good portion of neurological development, as well. We have always prioritized sleep in our home since the children were infants. We struggled with sleep so badly with Grayson, that we have never again taken it for granted. I saw first hand what the lack of sleep can do to a human, and it's not pretty. All joking aside, be sure your kids and you get the proper amount of quality sleep, as it is in large part responsible for your functioning state of mind. If you aren't well rested with good quality sleep, the deficits can be subtle initially, but they will catch up with you, especially if your sleep deficit is chronic.

Lack of sleep will affect emotional intelligence, as well as higher-level cognitive abilities. It even increases susceptibility to infections, which has probably been evident at one time or another in your past. You may recall a time when you stayed out much later than usual and just happened to come down with some sort of illness shortly after, a cold or the flu. As a homeopath, I have been trained to make sure sleep is addressed first and foremost, because even with the proper remedies and treatment, if sleep is suffering, so is the person.

It's possible to reduce or even eliminate many chronic symptoms by working out the sleep issues. It is not only important for children, but the adults who care for children must also be sure to get enough rest. It's hard enough navigating through some days, add sleep deprivation to the list and you become a ticking time bomb.

Here are a few practical tips for a better slumber:

- Keep a schedule, this helps to regulate your body's circadian rhythm.
- Practice a relaxing bedtime routine, especially with the kiddos. This routine will prepare their body for the pending zzzz's.
- Keep it calm, it's even a good idea to keep lighting and sounds low and soothing for the hour before heading to bed.
- Keep the temperature cooler at night and make sure to eliminate any light sources in the bedroom.
- I highly recommend a sound machine. We have used them religiously with our children and ourselves, we even travel with them. They drown out sounds that can cause startling during sleep.

If all else fails and your child is struggling with sleep (which means you are too) and you have established that nothing serious is contributing to the problem, try a sleep training book like "The Baby Whisperer Solves all Your Problems." It worked wonders for us when Grayson was struggling to get out of some bad habits that were initiated when he was not feeling well.

SPIRITUAL ENHANCEMENT

How to become more spiritually enhanced is going to look different for every person. I found that for me, spiritual enhancement wasn't as much about seeking, as it was about being open to the lessons embedded in my experiences. Many associate the word "spiritual" with religion and this confusion often sends some people running the other direction. Whether we recognize it consciously or not, everything we think and do, how we respond to trauma and excitement, what moves us to cry and laugh, all of our self-talk, and even why we choose to lean towards certain healing modalities, all has it's roots in our spiritual being. The conditioning of our upbringing, whether religious or not, is a spiritual experience. Life is a spiritual experience.

The definition of spirit according to the Oxford Dictionaries is

> *"The nonphysical part of a person that is the seat of emotions and character; the soul: 'we seek a harmony between body and spirit'."*

Synonyms of spirit are: soul, psyche, mind, ego, pneuma, (inner) self, inner being. So you see, we can go nowhere and do nothing without our spirit in tow, therefore, our spirit is intimately connected to our behaviors!

It is when we bring our spiritual body into consciousness that we begin to label the experience, thereby identifying with it. For some, this looks like organized religion, for others it has its own self-imposed boundaries and ideals. Either way, this is a journey that demands respect and patience. Although I began to become consciously aware of my own spiritual journey when Grayson was a toddler (mainly because I decided it needed my focus), it had only touched the tip of the iceberg. In hindsight, I have since concluded that my journey actually began at my own conception. The course of my life carried me to this point, with purpose, every painful and joyful experience. Becoming consciously aware of this journey has enabled me to be an active participant, thereby enriching my life with direction which colored my path to purpose, and has exposed insight as well as outreach opportunities. Since every experience is an active part of your spiritual journey, please use grace and compassion in your self-reflection and remember that failure ignites growth.

SURROUND YOURSELF WITH SUPPORTIVE, LIKE-MINDED PEOPLE

Contrary to popular belief, genetics don't guarantee being born into a family of like- minded people, nor is it necessary. Healthy skepticism is a good form of checks and balances. A strong foundation (root chakra) will keep you grounded in your truth and merely by living and believing in yourself, you will naturally influence others. Some will join you in your quest, while others will just watch from a distance. Be prepared for your open lifestyle changes to inflame some people too. Remember that our state of mind carries it's own vibration. Some will resonate with you and may actually be drawn to you by sheer harmonic entrainment and some will completely resist the disruption to their own frequency. Just know that their story doesn't have to be like yours. Mutual respect can allow a lot of growth for both in this situation. Kill 'em with kindness is my motto here.

If you are surrounded by people who regularly emit harsh energy or constant criticism of your belief system, it may require you to live against the grain, which is quite like swimming against the current constantly. And I promise you, this will become tiring, it won't be long before you are even questioning yourself just to end this tiring struggle.

Don't feel bad if you feel the need to create some space between you and those who just can't seem to respect your choices. But please do it with kindness, otherwise you have joined their frequency rather than influencing them with yours. Or, as you may have heard others say, you have stooped to their level, not in ego, but in frequency. No one is on the exact same journey, no one.

Even our young children have their own unfolding stories. We must respect others' journeys, if we expect them to respect ours. We are not going to see eye to eye with everyone. I encourage you to find your tribe, the people you are in alignment with. This level of support can come from local groups and/or social media groups. It will deepen your experiences and you will find comfort in the mutual bonds you develop with those who truly get you. This support is indispensable when you find yourself in a situation where you need advice that aligns with your current lifestyle. I couldn't have made it this far without my tribe.

TOUCH

As infants, our children naturally receive a lot of touch, it's built into infancy due to general care and honestly, who doesn't love to cuddle an infant, right? It triggers lots of great feel-good hormones. But as we get older, it's not uncommon to experience less touch.

Once we start walking, touch goes down significantly, and even more so as children turn into teenagers. It's so easy to forget to keep the act of touch alive. Touch is essential to our being and can be easily brought back into our lives with hugs, massage, cuddling, and even pats on the back or a tussle of the hair for those hard-to-touch teens out there. Some kids really crave roughhousing which is a legitimate form of touch. If the roughhousing is excessive, consider adding in more random touch, and remember that a craving for constant firm pressure (which may surface as roughhousing) can be a symptom of sensory processing disorder. Touch and smile at your family members often!

TUNING FORKS AND SINGING BOWLS

We just love the immediate vibratory lift from using tuning forks and singing bowls. It's instantaneous! They are great to use during meditation or even physically on the body in coordination with the effected chakra(s).

Our younger son is considerably effected by large crowds, he tends to take on the energy around him, good and bad unfortunately. Carrying a tuning fork (heart or angel frequency) in my purse offers him a quick pick-me-up and energy rebalance and it can be done quickly in the car or anywhere, for that matter.

Kids love to play with tuning forks and will resonate with the frequency they need, so feel free to buy a set and leave it out for all to use or play with. Healing with music is a fabulous thing to research.

VAGUS NERVE ACTIVATION

Think of the vagus nerve as the super highway connecting the brain and the gut. The vagus nerve is the longest nerve in the autonomic nervous system and while it's known for it's critical roles in controlling the heart, lungs and digestive tract, it was once thought to be controlled by the brain, yet we've since learned that for every one message going from the brain to the gut, there are nine traveling from the gut to the brain! Messages can be transmitted from the gut to the brain in seconds, releasing hormones into the blood stream on demand. Perhaps you've heard the term "the gut-brain connection", that "gut feeling" or more technically labelled as the "brain-gut axis." This is referring to the vagus nerve and it's feedback loop which can produce either positive or negative outcomes.

The vagus nerve is the main component of the parasympathetic nervous system which oversees the bodily functions listed above, but also our mood and immune system. You may have heard of "rest and digest," which is associated with the parasympathetic nervous system. Activation of the vagus nerve has become the target of treatment for various psychiatric and gastrointestinal disorders, due to it's ability to inhibit cytokine production and modulate mood and anxiety disorders. People with neurodevelopment disorders often have low vagal nerve tone. Multiple studies and findings suggest that vagal nerve stimulation (VNS) enhances recovery from neurodevelopment disorders.

There is mounting research and support for a growing trend towards mental health care that uses bacteria which have a direct influence over mood and anxiety. This superhighway is the path by which those bacteria communicate with the brain. Beneficial bacteria have the uncanny ability to activate the vagus nerve resulting in mediating effects on the brain and behavior, but even more intriguing is that the vagus nerve may actually be able to differentiate between non-pathogenic and pathogenic bacteria inducing signals to release various biochemical mediators in response. So daily intake of beneficial bacteria has just taken on a whole new meaning. Do it for your vagus nerve.

There are numerous simple ways to stimulate the vagus nerve, many of which we do without even realizing it! Things like singing, humming, gargling, exposure to the cold, probiotics, meditation and exercise all activate the vagus nerve. Activation of the vagus nerve can increase vagal tone which is associated with positive emotions, healthy social connections and better physical health. Other ways to activate the vagus nerve, and this list is by no means, complete: sing, hum, chant, chew gum (healthy gum), gargle, meditate, yoga, TaiChi, fast intermittently, acupuncture, prayer, get massages often, use enemas, PEMF treatment on the neck, head and gut, drink cold water, dip the face in cold water or take cold showers. Surprisingly, gluten sensitivity has been shown to disrupt gut health resulting in reduced vagal tone. Reason 253 for avoiding gluten. Just kidding, I am not keeping count...yet.

The vagus nerve is influenced by breathing which is why focus on the quality of breath during practices like yoga, Tai Chi and meditation have such a profound effect on the mood. There is a simple technique I like to use for activating the vagus nerve which can be done anywhere, anytime and in a matter of minutes. Don't laugh, but I have also been known to put this on my calendar reminding me to take time during the day to activate my vagus nerve intentionally. This technique is also helpful in a pinch when stress overwhelms you. It's a modified version of deep breathing, focusing on extended exhales. I know its seems odd that your exhale count is longer than the inhale count, and most people teach deep inhalation breaths during stressful moments. The intent with deep breaths is to flood the blood with oxygen. In this case, the breathing pattern is specific to stimulating the vagus nerve. The ratio of counts you will use are 4:8, meaning you will take four seconds to inhale and a full eight to exhale. I like to use my fingers to keep track while I do this exercise for a few minutes. On the inhale, count 1-2-3-4, then exhale and count 1-2-3-4-5-6-7-8 and repeat, that's all! Easy enough to teach a toddler (as you count it out together).

A great product for stimulating the vagus nerve is called Sophia Flow by Sophia Nutrition. Dr. Klinghardt recommends this product with vagus nerve stimulation in mind, and is especially beneficial for those who have experienced mold toxicity. It is a cream containing brain-beneficial bacteria (Bifidobacteria and kefir grains) and phos-phatidylcholine which is vigorously rubbed into the vagus nerve before bedtime. You literally use a dot the size of a pea and even with three of us using it regularly, one jar lasts many months (at least five, maybe six). I have noticed a difference using this product, making it well worth the cost.

Fun fact about the vagus nerve is that laughing increases vagal tone, so laugh often!

VISION BOARD

A vision board is a visual method of focusing on what you want to see change in your life. Visualization is one of the most powerful mind exercises you can do. It's a bit like posting up a picture of your weight goal to work towards, but it can be used for everything and anything you want to see improve in your life. According to the book The Secret,

> *"The law of attraction is forming your entire life experience and it is doing that through your thoughts. When you are visualizing, you are emitting a powerful frequency out into the Universe."*[1]

Our family created a large vision board together, each with our own section of focus. A vision board creates a springboard for manifestation. It is a daily reminder to stay aligned with what you want, rather than what you don't want.

When you continue to focus on what you DO want, your natural tendency is to create that life by leaning towards activities and decisions that bring you closer to your goals. As Buddha said, *"What we think, we become."*

---

1. Rhonda Byrne, *The Secret*, Simon and Shuster (1994)

VITAMIN D

You might think this belongs in the "nutrition" category, and it does (and it is) if you need a vitamin D boost, but this time I am talking about getting outside! Nothing beats natural production of vitamin D. The best way to expose yourself to the rays of the sun and to avoid burning, is to start slow. In the Spring, start exposing more of yourself and your children's skin, as much skin as possible, to the early or late sun (before 11am and after 3pm) for very short spurts of time. Continue to increase your exposure over time, building up tolerance. Only 10-15 minutes of high-noon sun exposure is needed to produce all the vitamin D you need for the day. Vitamin D deficiency can be a contributing factor to some forms of skin cancer, but it is important to know how to properly expose your skin to the sun to avoid creating DNA damage. Vitamin D is also crucial to calcium absorption. If you live in the Northern Hemisphere where long days of sun is limited to a few short seasons in the year, or you tend to maintain a low vitamin D level, supplemental vitamin D3 might be helpful to carry you through the winter. Be sure to *always* pair vitamin D3 with vitamin K2, since both are required together for proper calcium metabolism.

Deficiency in vitamin K or an imbalance in D/K2 will cause calcium to accumulate in inappropriate places, resulting in symptoms like bone spurs, while causing systemic deficiency in calcium. Hypercalcemia is a condition where there is too much calcium in the wrong places and not enough in the essential places.

When it comes to testing, this is one test I highly recommend doing periodically. There are many at-home tests you can order online now, this being one of them. The test kit comes with a small spring-triggered lancet that pricks the finger. A simple blood spot is sent in for results.

WORDS HOLD POWER - EXPERIMENT

Throughout the book, I mention the importance of raising our vibration and how everything has its own vibrational thumbprint. Words are no exception, and to illustrate this, we duplicated an experiment that was initially demonstrated by the work of Dr. Masaru Emoto, who was a Japanese author of "the Hidden Messages in Water," and entrepreneur who said that human consciousness has an effect on the molecular structure of water.

My boys and I cooked organic white rice, let it cool briefly and then immediately transferred it into two different sterilized, identical glass jars with lids. One jar was labeled with the word "love" and the other was labeled with the word "hate." Each day, the boys and I picked up and spoke to the jars, according to their label. The hate jar received a lot of negative talk while the love jar received only loving comments. It was comical at first, to be talking to jars in this way, but what we quickly noticed is that it was actually painful and hard to say all the hateful things to the "hate" jar. Even using the words just for this experiment felt bad to us.

Within the first 24 hours, the "hate" jar of rice clouded up and became foggy while the "love" jar of rice remained nice and clear.

It wasn't long before we saw the first speck of mold in our "hate" jar, which continued to grow in size and location. This project spanned 60+ days, yet our "love" jar never developed any mold and the rice retained it's white color through the entire experiment, while the "hate" jar quickly grew mold and the color of the rice turned a dingy yellow.

What was even more interesting is how the "hate" jar's glass quickly turned foggy and remained that way throughout the experiment, while the "love" jar's glass remained clear.

We documented with daily photos to watch the progress over the span of the entire 60 days. It was astonishing how quickly the "hate" jar changed, while the "love" jar remained unaffected. Dr. Emoto's experiment contained one extra dimension to this experiment. He added a third jar of rice, which was ignored (neglect) and this jar rotted while his "hate" jar grew mold and his "love" jar fermented pleasantly like a fermenting food on the counter should.

If we apply this to our bodies, which are more than 70% water… and you can understand why loving kindness is essential to good health. Please think about the words you use not just with others, but even during your own self-talk! The global consequences of collective consciousness is also at play here. The environment we created in our little experiment can be duplicated on a much larger scale, involving the condition of our earth. Practicing loving kindness has the potential to change not just our lives, but our world. Please model what you'd like to see change around you. Change starts with you.

YOGA

During the thick of my awakening, yoga was my daily savior. Similar to my meditation experiences, I like to enhance yoga with coordinating music.

Yoga has a unique ability to invigorate the body while calming the mind. Many of the movements are designed to release stored energy very similar to chiropractic care so you can even focus on particular areas of concern, if you want. I found that I was also more inclined to meditate directly following yoga practice so it was a double-whammy.

There are many YouTubers who teach yoga, so now-a-days you don't even need to go to a studio or spend money for a trained yoga experience, but if you are a fan of the collective consciousness experience from being together with others drawing in the same energy, you may prefer to find a studio that suits your needs. Also, if you prefer hot yoga, the only way to get that experience is to go to a studio.

FOR THE HOME AND BODY

CONSIDERING the microbiome is in every cell of our body, everything we put on and in our bodies has the potential to influence our microbiome, which in turn influences our neurological health. Even the air we breath can aid in healing or harming us.

As you saw in the diagram in "Overflowing Buckets," in part I of the book, we must manage the incoming toxins if we want to keep our toxin load from overflowing. In this section you will learn more about the things we have going on around us that influence our total toxin load, as well as things we can do or use to improve our response to toxins.

CLEANING AND DISINFECTING

An easy and very inexpensive place to start cleaning up the toxins around your home is to change the way you clean, more importantly, change *what* you use to clean. Reducing these toxins in the home will also impact the earth, because everything we flush down a toilet, sink or tub, also ends up in our water table where it can effect our environment.

When we sit our little ones in a nice warm bath, imagine their pores opening up and absorbing whatever is in that water…do you want the bleach or chemical cleaner you just coated the tub with to enter your child's bloodstream? If you used it on the tub, it is doing just that!

The EPA ranks indoor air quality as a top five environmental risk to public health. EPA studies found indoor air pollutants were generally 2-5 times greater than outdoor pollution levels and in some cases, this soared to 100x greater! Many things contribute to this air pollution, like: poor ventilation, the use of air fresheners, chemical laden household cleaners, toxic paints, varnishes and furniture treated with fire retardants, mold biotoxins and so on. So, if you can work to reduce this burden in your environment, one step at a time, you will increase the quality of your indoor air.

There are many healthier products coming to the commercial market, but you must also be careful, because many of them advertise one thing and deliver another. I always use the Environmental Working Group website to help me navigate healthy options for the home and body. Making your own inexpensive bulk cleaning supplies is a great alternative to the commercial products and will be as pure as the ingredients you create them with.

My failsafe go-to cleaner for anything that requires disinfection is always food-grade hydrogen peroxide. It is by far, the most effective disinfectant out there.

Another staple in our home is Norwex. This company has stolen the market when it comes to healthy cleaning. Their microfiber products are all embedded with silver and the combination of the silver and microfiber is just brilliant. The microfiber locks onto dirt, wiping it away with ease and the silver destroys microbes. I once watched a UV light demonstration comparing the effectiveness of Lysol with Norwex. The Lysol left behind disgusting residue while the Norwex wiped the surface spotless in just a few swipes of the towel. They are great for the environment too, because they cut down on paper product use, bonus!

Another amazing cleaner for the home, which I am never without, is the use of environmental probiotics (see more about environmental probiotics in a separate category), which I like to spray around the house, as well as wiping down surfaces, so that the good bacteria continue to keep the environment clean for days. I especially like these products for: upholstered surfaces, closets, garbage cans, plants and bedding which can't easily be disinfected or wiped clean. A probiotic mist does just the trick. It even does a great job on the interior of our cars. Think of the many environmental toxins that hitch a ride with you in your car!

COOKWARE

The act of heating synthetic substances and metals for the purpose of cooking your food comes with much greater risk than many recognize. It's easy to take our cookware for granted, never thinking past the food itself. Studies are confirming that toxins can leach into food from the cooking surface of your cookware. Aluminum pots and pans are linked to Alzheimer's and dementia. Non-stick cookware made from polytetrafluoroetheylene (PTFE) breaks down into a chemical warfare agent known as PFIB, and a chemical analog of the WWII nerve gas phosgene. Poisons! The Environmental Working Group commissioned tests conducted in 2003 which showed that in just two to five minutes on a conventional stove top, cookware coated with Teflon and other non-stick surfaces could exceed temperatures at which the coating breaks apart and emits toxic particles and gases.

It took me a while to really fine tune my understanding of the cookware options out there. I've done a lot of research and experimenting with cookware. I went through multiple stages of understanding the materials. It started with stainless steel, which was better than the non-stick cookware I had previously used, but still not great, because lower quality stainless steel could have high nickel content (and Grayson tested off the charts for nickel). Then I discovered cast iron, which I thought was the best cookware since sliced bread, but it was soon brought to my attention that too much iron, especially inorganic forms of iron like the kind in cast iron cookware, is dangerous for the body, as well. It can cause infertility and hemorrhaging, as well as damaging the liver. Then I jumped on the Le Creuset bandwagon and sadly discovered that when the glaze surface gets scratched (which is inevitable if you have a man cooking in your kitchen) lead leaches from the damaged glaze. Another brand I have used is Xtrema ceramic cookware. I do love ceramic cookware, but again, there is the risk of damaged glaze releasing lead into the food and testing has confirmed lead in this brand as well. So it seems that no ceramic brands are truly lead-free unless they are brand-new and unharmed by utensils and wear.

I ultimately decided to look for the cleanest stainless steel I could find. With cookware it appears that we have to choose the lesser of the evils. Everything I read reiterated that buying stainless steel brands made in the USA is the best way to ensure safer levels of metals.

USA PAN is a family owned business in Kansas with all of the materials made right here in the USA.

All-Clad is another brand manufactured in the United States with high quality, full-ply stainless steel options, but keep in mind that they also carry other, cheaper collections , some even with toxic non-stick surfaces. 10% of their products are made in other countries, including China, so just be sure to research the collections fully before deciding on one.

360 Cookware looks like a wonderful USA-manufactured, high quality brand. I love that they offer stainless steel bake ware, which is really rare. They also carry very high quality flatware sets.

Unfortunately, in the case of cookware, *you get what you pay for* and cheaper collections are usually the result of cheaper materials.

What ever you choose, make sure you look at third party reviews and product testing. Anything with a glaze must be monitored regularly, because once the glaze is compromised, the materials from beneath the glaze can leach into your food.

EMR, EMF, RF, AND WIFI EXPOSURES

This is a broad topic and encompasses multiple considerations which are mentioned below, but it is also a topic not to avoid, because it is incredibly important! For sensitive individuals such as those with Autism, autoimmune disease and multiple sensitivities, this is something to take seriously, although there is no one that this doesn't effect. I'm going to repeat this for your benefit, there is NO ONE that this doesn't effect. The electro-hypersensitive population is just blessed with the ability to still react to what their body views as harmful. The "radiation" I am referring to when I say EMR relates to man-made electromagnetic radiation which was intro-duced into our environment as an unexpected byproduct of modern electricity.

Hundreds of studies have been conducted throughout the world and many informed doctors and independent researchers have made statements about their concerns on the health effects of this man-made bombardment of EMR. During the EMF Summit, guest speaker and pioneer in this field, Dr. Klinghardt said,

> *"Everybody exposed gets an altered consciousness, the same increase in cancer rates later in life, cardiovascular disease, neurological disease."*

His opening discussion at the EMF Summit was compelling! In the 1960's he was taught by his professors that through experimenta-tion using microwave radiation on people, it was discovered that 2.4 gigahertz frequencies is the ideal frequency to sterilize a whole population over 2 or 3 generations. It induces epigenetic damage to the systems making them less likely to be fertile. This is passed on to the offspring, who is then also blasted with radiation during their lifetime. In the 60's when this was being taught, this frequency was not being used. Now, all wireless applications use 2.4 gigahertz!! Interestingly, Russia and Iran use different frequencies! He went on to explain that for those with heavy metal toxicity, dispersed heavy metals in our bodies are actually like little antenna. They are receivers.

By decreasing the metals in the body, the body becomes less vulnerable to the environment. One cell phone call with the phone placed to your head can liberate 600x more mercury from amalgam fillings than would have otherwise been released. There are issues with gold crowns and titanium implants, as well. Dental revision must be part of the quest for health. The good news is that there are solutions for all of these concerns. Read on to learn about each type of EMF and ways to mitigate the effects.

There is promising clinical research suggesting that the use of herbal Phyllanthus Fraternus, also known as Chanca Piedra, is protective against the brain damage that manifests from EMF exposure. For more information, go to the "Supplementation" section of this Resource Guide.

EMF stands for electromagnetic frequencies and is the most commonly and interchangeably used term when it comes to the resulting frequencies surrounding electrical devices. Most devices contribute to more than one form of EMR though, so it's important to understand the various forms of radiation, how they are measured, and more importantly, how they can be reduced.

Extremely Low Frequency (ELF) are measured in terms of their electric and magnetic components. The electric field is related to the voltage in the conductor. Electric fields are present even if no current is flowing. For instance, a plugged-in lamp and the cord to it have an electric field, even if the lamp is not turned on. Electric fields are measured in V/m, or volts per meter. The magnetic field is generated by the current flowing through a conductor, and the currents can vary in strength. Magnetic field strength is measured in milliGauss (mG), which is 1/1000 of a Gauss. The lower the frequency, the longer the wavelength. The higher the frequency, the shorter the wavelength. The shorter the wave, the more power is in it.

As we move up the EM spectrum from the longer to the shorter wavelengths, we encounter first electrical power transmission, then radio, TV, radar/microwave, radiant heat/visible light, ultraviolet, x-rays and gamma rays. The frequencies at and below that of visible light are known as non-ionizing, and those above light as ionizing. At ionizing frequencies, the particles of radiation contain enough energy to eject electrons from atoms and molecules, leaving them electrically imbalanced, or ionized. Ionized molecules are highly reactive and can damage cells. As technology advanced and we began to use the higher frequencies, it was accidentally discovered that frequencies of about 27MHz (27 mega Hertz, or 27 million cycles per second) caused body heating.

Dr. Neil Cherry who was Associate Professor of Environmental Health at Lincoln University, New Zealand spent many years traveling around the world visiting universities and laboratories collecting published papers and speaking with the original researchers to put together data supporting rising concerns surrounding the health effects of EMR. In a summary report by Dr. Cherry, he concludes:

> *"Scientific studies at the cellular level, whole animal level and involving human populations, show compelling and comprehensive evidence that RF/MW exposure down to very low levels, levels which are a minute fraction of present "safety standards", result in altered brain function, sleep disruption, depression, chronic fatigue, headache, impaired memory and learning, adverse reproductive outcomes including miscarriage, still birth, cot death, prematurity and birth deformities. Many other adverse health effects have been found, predominantly cancer of many organs, especially brain cancer, leukemia, breast cancer and testicular cancer. Studies have also found that RF/MW exposed parents have more children with CNS [central nervous system] cancers and other health defects. These*

effects are consistent with genetic damage caused by RF/MW. Many scientific studies have found chromosome aberrations and DNA damage with RF/MW exposure, the first being published in 1959. Two primary biological mechanisms are linked to these effects, calcium ion efflux and melatonin reduction. With melatonin reduction, there is a rise in serotonin, which is associated with awakeness, alertness, anxiety, anger, rage and violence depending on the serotonin level, the person and the circumstances.

Hence, there is strong evidence that ELF and RF/MW is associated with accelerated aging (enhanced cell death and cancer) and moods, depression, suicide, anger, rage and violence , primarily through alteration of cellular calcium ions and the melatonin/serotonin balance."

As reported at an EMF conference:

"More than 100 epidemiological studies have shown an association between residential and occupational EMF exposure and many types of cancer. The association between EMF exposure and childhood cancer is especially strong. This scientific evidence led the 28 member panel convened by the National Institute of Environmental Health Sciences (NIEHS) to conclude on July 24, 1998, that extremely low frequency (ELF) electromagnetic fields should be regarded as possible carcinogens. The final vote of the panel was 19 to 9 in favor of categorizing ELF EMFs, such as those from power lines and electrical appliances, as possible carcinogens. The vote followed a year of exhaustive evaluation of the scientific literature, three multi-day symposia attended by many international scientists, and a final 10 day review and debate of the scientific and medical literature in a closed meeting in Minnesota."

In October 2002, a team of over 50 German medical doctors started the Freiburger Appeal. After seeing a dramatic rise in severe and chronic diseases, they have noted a clear temporal and spatial correlation between disease and exposure to microwave radiation. The appeal has since been signed by thousands of doctors. To quote:

"Out of great concern for the health of our fellow human beings do we – as established physicians of all fields, especially that of environmental medicine – turn to the medical establishment and those in public health and political domains, as well as to the public. We have observed, in recent years, a dramatic rise in severe and chronic diseases among our patients, especially:

- *Learning, concentration, and behavioral disorders (e.g. attention deficit disorder, ADD)*
- *Extreme fluctuations in blood pressure, ever harder to influence with medications*
- *Heart rhythm disorders*
- *Heart attacks and strokes among an increasingly younger population*
- *Brain-degenerative diseases (e.g. Alzheimer's) and epilepsy*
- *Cancerous afflictions: leukemia, brain tumors*

Moreover, we have observed an ever-increasing occurrence of various disorders, often misdiagnosed in patients as psychosomatic:

- *Headaches, migraines*
- *Chronic exhaustion*
- *Inner agitation*
- *Sleeplessness, daytime sleepiness*
- *Tinnitus*
- *Susceptibility to infection*
- *Nervous and connective tissue pains, for which the usual causes do not explain even the most conspicuous symptoms*

Since the living environment and lifestyles of our patients are familiar to us, we can see (especially after carefully-directed inquiry) a clear temporal and spatial correlation between the appearance of disease and exposure to pulsed high-frequency microwave radiation (HFMR), such as:

- *Installation of a mobile telephone sending station in the near vicinity*

- *Intensive mobile telephone use*
- *Installation of a digital cordless (DECT) telephone at home or in the neighborhood We can no longer believe this to be purely coincidence, for:*
- *Too often do we observe a marked concentration of particular illnesses in correspondingly HFMR-polluted areas or apartments*
- *Too often does a long-term disease or affliction improve or disappear in a relatively short time after reduction or elimination of HFMR pollution in the patient's environment*
- *Too often are our observations confirmed by on-site measurements of HFMR of unusual intensity.*

On the basis of our daily experiences, we hold the current mobile communications technology (introduced in 1992 and since then globally extensive) and cordless digital telephones (DECT standard) to be among the fundamental triggers for this fatal development."

A component of EMF results in measurable body voltage effects on humans and animals when they are standing in the field emitted by AC currents in electrical installations, cables, appliances, transformers, anything with a motor, overhead and ground cables and high-tension and other power lines. These fields can be detected as far as 6-8 feet around the source, meaning when you are simply standing in a room that contains electricity (not even counting the plugged in devices in the room) you would be in the field of housing wires when standing within 6-8 feet of any wall.

To compound matters, many rooms also contain plugged in appliances like clocks, lamps, radios, kitchen gadgets, and larger appliances like stoves, refrigerators, washers and dryers. Every one of these plugged in devices also emits EMF and magnetic frequencies, and depending on the device, possibly even RF as well! Body voltage from electricity can be detected with a body voltage meter, and this information can also be used to assist in the reduction of exposure for sleeping areas. Body voltage should be kept ideally under .010 V according to the Building Biology Evaluation Guidelines for sleeping areas. Our Building Biologist said that she would be happy with anything under 1V, which she said can be very hard to attain for most. At 2.5V, sleep disturbance and health consequences have been documented.

When we tested Grayson's body voltage while lying on his bed, the highest reading detected was 4.9V which was not surprising, because he was also the one person in our house who has had the most trouble falling asleep and waking unrefreshed, as well as often experiencing random bouts of anxiety and outbursts. To reduce body voltage from surrounding electrical sources, there are a few different tactics that can be used. For small reductions in exposure, all plugged in sources of electricity can be unplugged, or even better, use single port outlet switches that allow you to turn the source off at the outlet, thereby reducing the accumulative electrical fields. Nothing should be left plugged in when it is off, because the electricity is still being drawn into the wiring around the room and the effect on the wiring is accumulative. This only reduces numbers slightly though.

To really have an impact on Grayson's room, we needed to experiment with turning off breakers. Just turning off the breaker to the kitchen below his room (where ceiling fixtures require wires to run directly below Grayson's bed) dropped his body voltage to 2.1V! It is also important to watch how turning off breakers effects other rooms, because shunting the electricity can also increase the voltage by means of cancellation. For example, we had gotten Gavin's 1.8V reading down to .850V by just unplugging everything in his room, but turning off the breaker to his room actually increased the body voltage at his bed!

The lowest body voltage reading in Gavin's room resulted from just unplug his clock, radio and lamps. We use remote single port outlet switches that he can control at the touch of a button. When not in use, the item is turned off at the outlet completely by using his remote (which does cause a single burst of RF like a garage door opener). It's a brilliant device marketed to the elderly and the handicapped, but the effects it has on ambient EMF values renders it a wonderful solution for sensitive people too.

When you don't need your lights on during the day, you can have their power cut off at the outlet, and at night when you are sleeping, use a battery powered analog clock. Turn off the power to everything else while sleeping. If you are like us and you rely on noise machines for a peaceful night's rest, just run a shielded extension cord from the hallway outside of your room and keep the device further than 6-8 feet from your bed. We were able to reduce our master bedroom from 3.9V to 0.129V just by turning off the breaker to our bedroom! We noticed a considerable difference in our quality of sleep immediately. In fact, after the second night, Gavin actually woke us from a deep sleep at 9:30am. We never slept in that late, or heavily. Our bodies must have been enjoying the deep REM sleep that had been interrupted for years.

Magnetic Fields are measured in milligauss (mG) and sources which are the same as the EMF sources include: AC currents in electrical installations, cables, appliances, transformers, anything with a motor, overhead and ground cables and high-tension and other power lines, etc. Documentation from the government in the UK has referenced studies suggesting that there may be an increase in the risk of childhood leukemia at higher than usual magnetic field exposures. A simple PubMed search for "childhood leukemia and high-voltage" will result in dozens of study results, and this is only a sliver of the mounting evidence for the health consequences of EMR. Magnetic fields are most accurately measured with a Gauss meter. I once tested my "low EMF" blow dryer which came in at a shocking 38.8 mG on the high setting and 70 mG on the low setting. This was the reading from my low EMF blow dryer, I wondered what standard blow dryers are putting out. So, I grabbed my old blower dryer which happened to be a high end hair dresser's blow dryer and it tested higher than my meter actually goes! That means it was over 1000 mG or 1G.

If the wiring in homes is well-designed and properly executed, the background levels should be less than 0.3 mG. Faulty wiring can cause strong magnetic fields in areas of the house, sometimes whole rooms. We discovered through testing that we had an area like this in our home and of all places, in the kitchen. We spend most of our time in the kitchen! We identified faulty wiring related to the light fixture above our kitchen island and the field reading of 2.53 mG extended well beyond our island and all the way around it where we prep food and wash dishes. When the light was off, the reading was still elevated at 1.2 mG. Even more concerning was that because low-frequency fields pass through walls, Grayson's room (including where he slept), above this light fixture was slightly effected by the magnetic field, but only when that particular light was on.

Reducing faulty wiring involves an electrician and hopefully one who understands the dilemma beyond the fact that the fixture works when the light is switched on. There are multiple YouTube videos on the topic to help you understand more about what is going on with faulty wiring. Identifying hotspots in your house is an effective way to reduce unnecessary radiation exposures. Now, leaving lights on when they aren't needed takes on a whole new meaning! I used to worry about the energy consumption and the money spent unnecessarily lighting empty rooms, but the health consequences are much more concerning.

RF stands for radio frequencies (also known as microwave radiation) which are high frequency electromagnetic waves and as mentioned earlier, encompasses wireless and high-frequency signals that come from devices such as: cell phones, internet-enabled iPads and tablets, digital broadcasting, TVs, DECT telephones, cordless phones, two-way radios, satellite receiving dishes, pagers, fax machines, CD players and other digital equipment, baby monitors, cell towers, some electronic games, high frequency pest repelling units, fish finders, assistive listening systems and devices for the hearing impaired, security systems, microwave ovens, WiFi technology, Bluetooth-enabled devices and smart meters.

Even more concerning are the pulsed or periodic signals seen with devices like smart meters, cell phones, DECT and digital broadcasting, to name a few. Troubling news coming from a plethora of studies now says that just a few minutes of RF exposure can open calcium channel gates for several hours. Voltage gated calcium channels may exist in most, if not all, human cells, and play important roles in the activation of the immune system, muscle development and function and neuronal communication. Considering most people have their cell phones and other devices turned on 24/7, their cells never have time to recover.

The consequences of this are great. Triggering calcium channels to open also triggers a glutamate release. As discussed in an earlier chapter, elevated glutamate causes brain cell death. Although these frequencies are considered non-ionizing, meaning they can't directly break apart cell structures, there is an indirect downstream effect that does ultimately cause cells to be destroyed in the same way. These open calcium channels allow too much calcium in, which also creates oxidation resulting in little tiny holes in the blood brain barrier. Neurotransmitters are able to leave the cells, and heavy metals, pollution, bacteria, viruses, etc. can enter more easily. The immediate observable effects on the person could be depression, anxiety and neurological effects, among other things. For teens with depression, I would highly recommend reviewing exposure to RF sources like cell phones and Bluetooth devices.

Other long term effects associated with abnormal calcium channel function, according to the latest research, include a growing number of diseases like immunodeficiency, muscular dystrophy and neurological diseases such as Alzheimer's Disease. It seems fitting that there is a steep rise in depression along with increased RF exposures from multiple sources. Many studies have confirmed the above and are now considered common knowledge within the industry.

I would make this a high priority with a child on the spectrum, as it has been suggested that the calcium metabolism is a big part of the

Autism presentation. As a possible means of support and preven-tion, I would recommend considering the use of cell salts that regu-late calcium metabolism in an attempt to mitigate the effects. Cell salts involved in the metabolism of calcium are Calcarea Fluor (cal-cium fluoride), Calcarea Phos (Calcium phosphate) and Silicea (Sili-ca). These are the same cell salts recommended for the treatment of osteoporosis which is a disease associated with calcium metabolism problems. Using them daily in the 6x to 12x potency can be taken for months at a time very much like you would take a supplement.

As if this isn't enough, RF radiation also has the capacity to cause cancer. In May of 2011, The WHO/International Agency for Research on Cancer (IARC) classified radiofrequency electromag-netic fields as possibly carcinogenic to humans (Group 2B), based on an increased risk for glioma, a malignant type of brain cancer, asso-ciated with wireless phone use. With the growing number of cell towers and antennae in neighborhoods, it is wise to check out anten-nasearch.com to find out how many of these structures are within a 4 mile radius of your home. Sadly, it is becoming less feasible to find homes without nearby towers and antennas and even from nearby neighbors! We personally have radiation entering our house from an audible (via an RF meter) detected device from one side, and from the other side we have ambient measurements of radiation from a nearby cell tower! It has been suggested that if you can see a cell tower from your home, it can also "see" you, meaning you are in it's direct line of fire.

The challenge with my personal situation is that we can not block the signals, because they are coming from either side of our home and the signal literally blankets our entire house. Putting any sort of fabric or blocking material on one wall of a room just bounces it back into the room from the exposure on the other side.

So the solution for this sort of scenario is to use radiation blocking mesh fabric canopies over the bed. They block radiation from all around and provide safe sleeping quarters, at minimum. Some situations will also require an additional piece of blocking material beneath the bed, but testing can confirm if this is necessary or not. I prefer to leave the bottom of the bed open from radiation blocking whenever possible, because we do need the frequencies of the earth and blocking it entirely may have counterproductive consequences. Having a canopy offers a safe place to take a quick retreat from the onslaught of this radiation when desired. Think of the number of pregnant women and infants who could benefit from something like this.

DE is dirty electricity (also known as electrical line noise), which appears to be less understood, but is equally as concerning as the rest of the electrical exposures listed above. DE is created by many electronics, appliances, energy-efficient lights, and other devices that run on electricity. The more devices plugged in, the higher the DE becomes in a home. It was only discovered to be a health problem in 1997 or 98 and is measured in milliVolts (mV) or microamps. The goal is to reduce dirty electricity in building wiring to 100mV or lower, where electrical hypersensitive people feel best.

Electricity expert, Dave Stetzer who is also responsible for training building biologists in North America, brought many published, peer-reviewed studies to my attention showing that dirty electricity has been discovered to have direct adverse biological effects on humans and animals. For example, blood sugar changes in direct response to dirty electricity within 20 minutes, and within 8 hours of exposure, the pH in saliva changes and neurotransmitters (especially dopamine) are effected.[1] Lighting dimmer switchers are especially concerning and are an easy fix with a simple $3.50 electrical box replacement. LED lighting creates dirty electricity and fluorescent (CFL) light bulbs not only send DE along the electrical wires, but it radiates through space, putting approximately 27 microamps into your body within a few feet of the fixture! The National Institutes of Environmental Health Sciences (NIEHS) determined that anything over 18 microamps is associated with an increased risk of cancer. 60 microamps are enough to stop a dog's heart and just 80 microamps will stop a human's heart, so you can see how significant these exposures can be, how little it takes to create consequential damage!

Thankfully, it is a fairly simple task to use wire conditioning filters to reduce these numbers, but unfortunately, there is also DE in the air surrounding electrical devices like CFL and LED light bulbs, dimmer switches, inverters, switch mode power supplies, computers, electronics, plasma TVs, variable speed motors, phone chargers, computer monitors, digital clocks and more. There are a handful of different DE reducing filters on the market, although some of the more common brands aren't actually recommended by electrical engineers who are also Building Biologists. The technology differs between capacitative filters and non-capacitative line conditioners. Most of the capacitative filters create a sort of a dam, where the power load sits, trying to get through the dam, and it can require a bit of effort to reroute the line noise, thereby resulting in added reactive frequencies to the power lines and indirectly causing an increasing magnetic field. Since filters require that they carry the power they are filtering, it would be best to use a device that captures and dissipates the dirty electricity rather than trying to harness it. The results of this type of device enables a broad range of frequency conditioning without adding anything to the wires. We were impressed at how quickly our numbers came down with just a few non-capacitative line conditioners put into outlets beside our electrical panel in the basement. Since some filtering devices cause magnetic fields to increase, be sure to test the location where you install the filters. The good news about magnetic fields (as long as they are isolated to the filter) is that they generally drop off quickly with distance. If there is faulty wiring in the home producing strong magnetic fields, this should be resolved *before* using filters since it can magnify the problem.

To monitor DE in the air around devices you can simply turn on an old AM radio (be sure not to use a new one with static reducers built into it) and set it between stations so you are hearing static. Then walk around your house and as you put the radio near devices that emit DE, you will hear the static change to higher pitched frequencies, some quite disturbing. The best way to manage these items is to unplug them when they aren't in use, but if the device serves a valuable function, like our HiTech Air Reactor, which runs 24/7, it should be used away from people whenever possible.

DC Magnetic fields are the result of steel components in furniture like beds, mattresses, boxsprings, sofas, appliances and building materials. The frequencies cause the metal to become magnetized. We avoid metal in our beds for this very reason. When we replaced Grayson's mattress, we knew we would eventually have to replace his boxspring too, but incidentally we forgot this little detail until we were trying to figure out why his AC body voltage was remaining very high on his bed. In hindsight, I realized why he was also getting a magnetic field around the lower half of his bed. Metal in beds is a big problem since this is where our body needs time and space to repair itself from the daily onslaught of toxins and EMR. Infants are regularly put to sleep in cribs lined with metal grids within inches of their bodies and then we turn on the baby monitor for our own peace of mind, not even recognizing the noxious fields we just surrounded our precious babies with! It's no wonder they often don't sleep well in their own beds.

5G - It has not been fully deployed in most cities (as of this writing in 2019-20), but there are cities embarking on beta trials currently. 5G technology is a form of mixed frequencies that will require small antennas to be installed in front of houses. One tower will need to be installed approximately ever 6-10 houses. The cell phone industry hasn't even committed to this technology yet, and there is word that they really don't want to go this direction, but the real problem will be all of the wireless devices brought into the home that will have this technology built into them. It will saturate your environment with constant EMF bathing. We are already massively overexposed by all of the wireless and Bluetooth devices found in homes like Roku and Apple TV, Smart TVs, wireless thermostats, and more. Adding 5G to the mix will be like EMF on steroids. To give you an idea of the amplitude of 5G, let's compare the frequencies with our current cell phone technology. 4G is 200-300Hz (cycles/second) and 5G ranges from 10MHz (that's 10,000,000Hz or 10 million cycles/second) to 300GHz (1GHz is 1 billion cycles/second!) Even if you move these devices away from you, say you decide to store your router in the garage, (which is a great start because it creates distance from the source), the minute you put your laptop on your lap and turn it on to connect with your router, you have just invited the electro-pollution into your lap!! The solution is to avoid having these devices in your house, period. Use some of the well-made, reasonably priced meters from a source like lessEM-F.com to measure your home so you can make educated decisions about your exposures. See some of the other headings under this topic for solutions to WiFi and Bluetooth. Also know that even your cell phone can be wire connected to an ethernet adapter for internet access while in airplane mode!

As with anything else, there will be varying effects when it comes to exposure reactions. EVERYONE is effected, but not everyone shows immediate signs of how EMF is effecting them individually. Reactions can also be accumulative and take years to show up, and it might require detective work to uncover the connection between the illness and the cause. Perhaps the timing of your Smart Meter installation tells you something about a new set of symptoms, or when you handed your child his first cell phone, his sleep began to suffer and you thought it was just because he was staying up too late. Next thing you know, he is moody and impulsive more frequently than he was before the phone.

Now that children are being born into this world with so much electro-pollution, it will become harder and harder to draw these types of conclusions. We are all saturated in it regularly if we aren't taking steps to mitigate our exposures. Sometimes it's hard to tell even when someone is reacting directly to the exposure until you eliminate it and then re- expose them to the source.

We lived in a house very near power lines when Grayson was born, so after he regressed into Autism, and we began researching its potential effects on health, we ultimately decided to move. I actually became pregnant with our younger son while still living there, and we have discovered that he is extremely emotionally effected by WiFi and close contact with handheld devices. It wasn't until we eliminated WiFi in our house (just to live healthier), then exposed him to WiFi elsewhere, that we were able to truly identify a severe reaction to it.

It has been established through studies, that there is a neurotransmitter response along with white matter development within the brain directly related to exposure from many different forms of technology. Under this umbrella, there are varying degrees of solutions to address exposure, and the degree of reaction is likely to control your depth of resolution. Regardless of whether you or a loved one experiences a direct reaction, studies are pointing to a fairly high level of concern as our technology develops, exposing us more and more consistently to low, high and pulsed frequencies throughout our environment. Since we homeschool our boys and spend a lot of time in our home, I've taken the approach that we will reduce as much exposure as possible, without moving off the grid entirely. The solutions we have adopted have proven to be useful for our family, and they include addressing the following:

Baby monitors
The newer baby monitors are utilizing the same technology as cell phones and there is growing concern about exposing babies to this form of radiation, especially during sleep which is when the body regenerates, heals and develops. Please also consider your baby's bed design and mattress, because adding metal to their sleep space magnifies body voltage and EMR. If you would still like to use a baby monitor, look for the older monitors that use the longer antenna rather than the short stubby antennas or use EMR reducing products that can be found under "EMR reducing supplies" in the website listings at the end of this book.

Blue-light blocking eye glasses

Light controls our wake-sleep circadian rhythms. In nature, we are exposed to the light spectrum. Blue light as a stand-alone exposure, which is emitted from screens of all kinds, suppresses melatonin production. By using blue-light blocking glasses, you can reduce the impact screens have on your circadian rhythm. Part of the problem with LED lighting (aside from the DE and EMR exposures) is that they emit high levels of blue light, which also messes with our circadian rhythm. Considering how important effective sleep is to our health, wearing blue-light blocking glasses during screen time is an easy way to tone down the effects from screens, especially if you need to use a device close to slumber-time or you like to watch TV before going to bed.

Cell phones

This can encompass an entire book on it's own, but quite simply, cell phones are incredibly concerning, especially for children. According to the Environmental Working Group, childrens' brains absorb twice the amount of cell phone radiation as adults' brains. Dr. Mercola shared images of brain scans of people using cell phones against their heads. The difference between adults and children was astonishing. It's bad enough that there is brain exposure to radiation during every single call, but in adults, that radiation remains fairly contained to the side of the head the phone is on. In children (up until about the age of 20) that same radiation is absorbed by the ENTIRE brain!

A study conducted by researchers from Indiana University, the University of Eastern Finland, the University of Campina in Brazil and the Institute of Experimental Pathology, Oncology and Radiology in Kieve, Ukraine found that radio frequency radiation used by cell phones and other wireless devices causes a metabolic imbalance known as oxidative stress. In 2011, the International Agency for Research on Cancer officially classified radio frequencies as a "possible carcinogen," which came a year after the international interphone study found that people who used a cell phone for ten years were 40% more likely to develop brain tumors. This risk was 400% higher in those who started using phones before the age of 20.

Thankfully, there are solutions to reducing cell phone radiation exposure, because cell phones aren't going anywhere anytime soon! One way to ensure reduced radiation to the head is to use speakerphone, but let's face it, we don't all want every call to be broadcast to everyone around us, so when you do need privacy, an air tube (notice I didn't say Bluetooth) device will conduct sound waves to the head, rather than EMF or RF. Bluetooth devices add another layer of radiation exposure. There are also radiation protective cases for carrying your phones.

Exposure to parts of the body is of great concern, as now there is repeated evidence of people developing cancer where they store their phones against their body. I see a lot of women putting their cell phones in the bra or shirt, this is considerably concerning due to the proximity of sensitive breast tissue and the prevalence of breast cancer.

Men who carry their phones in their pockets also must consider radiation exposure to their hips and genitals. Women should also consider how close their purse holds the phone to their body. The more distance you can create between yourself and your phone, the better. SAR (specific absorption rates) values are tested using set distances. A good radiation-blocking case can reduce exposure significantly. I would still recommend keeping cell phones a good distance from any body parts on a regular basis since no shielding device is 100% protective.

Our Building Biologist did a demonstration with my husband and I when she was doing an assessment of our home. My husband had been using the paired Bluetooth setting in his car, mistakingly thinking it was the best way to be hands-free while avoiding brain exposure to the RF radiation of his cell phone. She had us sit in his car with my husband's cell phone off. She turned on her meter while we turned on the car. As soon as the car came on, the pulsed readings were astonishing. They frequently reached 2.4uW/cm2 and higher as the Bluetooth was searching for the device. Even without the phone on, the radiation was very high. To complicate matters, using an RF device of any kind in a car exposes the driver and passengers to bouncing frequencies, which literally bounce around inside the metal frame of the car, magnifying exposure. It is never a good idea to leave a cell phone on inside of a car! Our Building Biologist said that this is THE worst exposure she often measures. She also told us a story about her brother in law who developed cancer at his hip, in the exact spot where he carries his cell phone. Sadly, this isn't the first time I've heard of stories like this and I'm sure, it won't be the last, either.

I am a huge advocate for cell-phone safety, especially for our youth. I once recorded a video using my Acousticom 2 microwave (RF) meter at the wall directly behind where our Smart Meter was installed. Then I took my cell phone out of airplane mode to show people how much worse our cell phones can be than our Smart Meters, depending on how we use them. This is the Facebook post I shared with that video:

> "I just want to put this out there. Like others, I'm not a fan of Smart Meters and I would most definitely opt out if I could. We take precautions like avoiding sitting near it and we use EMF canopies to protect the sleeping environment. We also have a Smart Meter guard, which is effective at reducing the radiation exposure. BUT, what we really need to be putting our attention on is our cell phones, which emit constantly when they are on, especially if you leave your Bluetooth, location and WiFi options activated. So, this video shows you first the wall on the other side of our Smart Meter. My cell phone is in airplane mode at first. Then I switch my phone out of airplane mode and you will see the meter leap into the red zone, which it never once reached with the Smart Meter alone, not even for the multiple minutes I watched it before recording. Keep in mind, my Smart Meter is covered with a Smart Meter Guard.

So people, if you are wearing your phones on your body all day long (or at all for that matter), the Smart Meter is the least of your worries. Cover your Smart Meter, it works. Now let's talk about that cell tower you wear on you hip all day, keep your cell phone in airplane mode anytime you are carrying it near your body. If you don't deactivate your Bluetooth, location and WiFi settings, it's just as good as being on. Do you really want your babies getting zapped with this cancer causing radiation? PLEASE don't give your babies cell phones to play on. Even in airplane mode, the screen is triggering neurotransmitter imbalance, setting up chemical dominance for addiction.

As I wrote this post, my phone was in airplane mode. I will place my phone on a flat surface, turn it on, hit the "share" button from a distance and walk away from it until it posts. These are the habits we need to be modeling and demanding from our youth. If they can't display safe habits with a phone, they aren't mature enough to have one! Would you give your child a driver's license at 8,10 or even 12 just because it's convenient for you? Make it about safety first and nothing else. There is no shame in taking away the keys if your child is displaying unsafe driving habits."

I often compare cell phone use with getting a driver's license, because I am adamant that children and adolescents should not have cell phones until they can consistently show maturity in their usage safety habits. In order to expect and demand cell phone safety from our kids, we must model it. This is what I would recommend modeling and teaching our youth about cell phone safety:

- Use a radiation reducing case (I recommend testing them, since some actually increase radiation output).
- Keep all tracking and notification settings turned off (WiFi, Bluetooth, and Location), especially when the phone is in close proximity to the body.
- Turn off notifications that aren't absolutely necessary. Each notification sends a signal to the phone. If you hear dinging, you are experiencing a radiation burst.

- Never use the Bluetooth connection in vehicles where the signal can bounce around becoming magnified.
- Keep phones in airplane mode when being carried against the body, while riding in vehicles and whenever they aren't in use. Even if you have to use the GPS, you can locate the route and then turn the phone onto the airplane mode and it will continue to provide guidance, unless you change your route; in which case turning it back on temporarily will reset the directions, updating the route, then you can switch the phone back into airplane mode again.
- When switching the phone out of airplane mode or turning it on, place the phone onto a surface nearby and keep a safe distance while all of the notification updates are completed.
- Use speakerphone or an air tube headset for phone calls (or use texting) and keep the phone away from your body during the call by putting it onto a surface nearby or in a bag or purse. Phones emit less radiation when using the text feature.
- If you absolutely have to make a private phone call and you don't have your headset nearby, keep the phone at least a 1/2" away from the head for a very brief call.
- Use a stylus pen rather than your finger.
- Try to use your phone when the signal is stronger (there are more service bars) because the radiation is greater when the signal is weak.
- Never keep your phone on your nightstand or under your pillow at night, instead, choose a common place away from your bed to store and recharge your phone.

Clocks and electronics on night stands

Keep them at a distance of at *least* 24 inches from the head/body to reduce the exposure to EMF, magnetic, RF (in enabled clocks) and dirty electricity radiation. Even better, unplug them entirely and use battery powered analog clocks (The LED causes DE radiation both in the wiring and around the device).

Cordless phones

Dr. Dietrich Klinghardt once said that having a cordless phone in your bedroom is like having a 747 jet engine running in your room. That is how much radiation these things give off. I thought I was doing my family a favor by purchasing a low-radiation cordless phone that was advertised as having an eco-setting and supposedly didn't give off any radiation when it was on standby and very little when it was in use. Upon testing with professional equipment by my Building Biologist, it was discovered that my cordless phone was emitting high levels of pulsed RF radiation constantly, at 5.4uW/cm2 even feet from the phone! Anything over 0.1uW/cm2 is considered an extreme anomaly. I thought I was eliminating my RF radiation by avoiding my cell phone throughout the day, when I was actually exposing myself to constant high radiation against my head every time I took a phone call from our cordless house phone. I immediately invested in a corded phone!! Never looking back. I combine long phone cords with a CordPro and an air tube head set so I can completely avoid the head set all together.

Dimmer switches

The most common source of dirty electricity and the easiest to mitigate. Dimmer switches create massive magnetic fields when the associated lights are turned on, both around the switch itself, and around the lights connected to the switch. Our dining room chandelier was on a dimmer switch, because I loved the ambiance of a dim dinner event, but once I realized the cost at which this ambiance came, I quickly swapped out the dimmer switch with a standard light switch. To compensate for the bright light of the chandelier, I swapped out the bulbs for lower wattage bulbs and added a few smaller light fixtures to the outside perimeter of the room (which are of course on outlet switches so they can be turned off at the outlet). It worked to recreate a softer ambiance without the harmful magnetic fields.

EarthCalm

This is one of many EMF home protection devices. It is hard to say if one is more effective than another, especially now that more are showing up on the radiation- reduction scene. I chose this product years ago when it was one of the few products being offered, so I am not promoting the product itself as much as the idea of an option in the science behind the product.

Mirror Resonance Technology (MRT) uses the Schumann Resonance, or the resonance of the earth, to reduce the impact of EMFs in your home's wiring. EarthCalm doesn't actually reduce or block the EMFs in the home, instead it uses the Schumann Resonance to ground the inhabitants, reducing the impact of the EMFs your home emits around you. The device uses your electrical wiring to send the grounding frequency of the earth throughout the whole house, engulfing you in this healing frequency. And why do we need to reduce the impact our electrical system has on our health? According to EarthCalm's research:

> *"Unfortunately, the AC electrical system in our homes runs on 50 or 60 Hz, which is in the same range as our body's own resonant frequency. For instance, our brain resonates at around 8 Hz. Because our body's resonant frequency is so close to our home's electrical system, resonance is established between our body and the house electricity, allowing energy to be transferred from the electrical wiring and appliances into our body's nervous system.*

> *This foreign energy knocks ions out of their proper position in the cell and interferes with cell metabolism. This phenomenon accounts for deficiencies in calcium (contributing to arthritis, anxiety), lithium (depression, schizophrenia), and potassium (Alzheimer's). In addition, EMFs from our AC electrical system induce biologically meaningless currents in our nervous system and brains. (In a sense, EMFs are like advertisements that interrupt our thinking.) We subconsciously receive meaningless information about how our appliances are working.*

This energy exchange, which can certainly be described as a subtle attack, generates stress hormones in the body, which in turn slowly erode the immune system and contribute to the many immune deficiency diseases that are common today."

There is a striking similarity between the effects of our electrical systems and some of the things we are seeing in Autism and PANDAS/PANS, isn't there? At any rate, since EMFs cannot be seen, heard, tasted or touched, I consider the product a valuable asset to our home. And how do we know if a product like this is working, according to the EarthCalm website,

"the only way to measure the effectiveness of EarthCalm products is to measure the reduction of stress in your body. This can be done by measuring blood pressure, reduction of headaches, better sleep, reduction of hyperactive symptoms in children, etc. Many people notice the reduction of tension right away.

Others need to note reduction in symptoms of stress over time."

All I can say is that we sleep and feel better at home than anywhere else. Since only one device is needed for the entire house, it's worth the shot that it might be working.

Hand-held electronic devices

Depending on the device, there is a whole host of issues with unsafe exposures related to handheld devices like tablets and phones. Hand-held devices bring EMR directly into the hands of little ones (and big ones). I cringe every time I see an infant playing with a parent's cell phone or iPad. The EMR on these devices is very strong, *especially* when they are plugged into the wall. Microwave radiation from iPads can be very high, especially while downloading content from the internet. When charging, iPads can also expose users to unusually high voltage levels from electric fields. To add to matters, it's not just the EMF from the devices that is troubling, it's also the WiFi resulting in pulsed RF.

Our younger son experiences changes in behavior with extended use of any handheld devices, so we aim to reduce exposure at all costs,. However, I do recognize that technology is a part of the world he will grow up in, so we have put some techniques of reducing exposure into practice, while also merely limiting his exposure in general. When he uses a handheld device, he uses a stylus pen, so his finger isn't directly activating the screen and we never allow use while the device is plugged into the wall. I always turn the WiFi off (on the device itself) when it isn't in use. Crystals such as quartz and fluorite can also reduce the effects of the EMF exposure from these electronic devices.

As if this isn't enough, there is one more major contributor to poor behavior following handheld device usage. Dopamine! Dopamine is a neurotransmitter that participates in the control of the pleasure systems of the brain. Scientists have discovered that the use of devices like cell phones, tablets and computers release dopamine, leading to the potential for addiction. This increase in dopamine is responsible for the behavior shifts seen in the more sensitive kids who crave electronic time. We all wear blue light blocking eyeglasses while using any electronic devices with screens, even the TV. The blue light disrupts melatonin production while increasing dopamine levels which is tied to addiction. It doesn't make screen-time 100% safe by any means, but every little bit helps, especially if you want to continue to enjoy the benefits of handheld devices while reducing the risks.

Microwave ovens

A microwave oven typically emits roughly 100-500 milligaus in EMFs from four inches away and I once tested ours, it continued to emit EMR clear across the kitchen, suggesting that perhaps the seal was broken on the door, although there was nothing visibly wrong with the door. This invisible damage in microwave doors will usually go undetected since the average person hasn't considered testing their microwave for radiation exposure. Considering how many microwaves are installed directly above the stove in newer homes, at head level, this exposure is extremely dangerous.

Besides the radiation exposure to the people in the kitchen, microwaves alter food so that it is unrecognizable by the body. It alters the food's chemical structure by forcefully tearing apart the molecules, causing deformity. A compounding concern with heating food in plastic, which is often the case when reheating food in a microwave, is that it leaches a multitude of chemicals into your food. Food should NEVER be heated in plastic of any kind, especially in a microwave. Our microwave merely served as storage until we had it professionally removed.

Shielding bed canopy

These sheer, mesh sleeping canopies are made with impregnated silver threads woven through nylon fabric and they provide 360 degrees of RF/microwave radiation protection. This is a simple (although costly) solution for circumstances out of your control, like nearby antennas or cell towers, Smart Meters and neighborhood WiFi blanketing your home. You can purchase them pre-made or buy the fabric to make your own, although I have not priced out a comparison. *It is important that these canopies are grounded!* If the canopy is not grounded (and some can't be) it will actually *increase* electrical fields around the bed, even though it is reducing radio frequencies. An ungrounded canopy should only be used if the body voltage in the bed is reduced to 0.18V during use, which is possible if you are turning off breakers to the room at night. Another good reason to own your own meters! We have one canopy that is grounded and another that cannot be grounded. I have personally measured the difference between the two. Thankfully, we can pull the ungrounded canopy up and away from the bed when the power is on in the room. When we go to sleep, we turn off the breaker to this room which eliminates the problem of increased electrical fields.

Smart Meter shield

Smart Meters are devices that are being placed onto houses (and businesses) by utility companies in order to comply with recent federal electrical grid changes. They transmit information to the utility company via radio frequencies. This is the same technology that is used by cell phones and studies are raising serious questions about this technology which has been demonstrated to be dangerous to the body. Smart Meters run around the clock and for more sensitive individuals, they can be highly problematic. If you have a smart meter, the readings can be over 100,000 mW/m2 (the threshold for concern is 10). Smart Meters are like having a cell tower on the side of your house. Some localities offer the option to opt-out, usually with a fee, some don't. Using Faraday cage technology, you can cover yours with a Smart Meter shield which blocks and absorbs 98-99% of the EMR. It's a very inexpensive solution for a potentially major problem.

When our house became the new owner of our first Smart Meter, I immediately hired a Building Biologist to assess our entire home. I had been considering a consultation for a while, but the Smart Meter put this on the front burner for me. So, I took the plunge. Turns out this is not uncommon, according to our consultant, who says a good number of her clients reached out to her because of their Smart Meter installations. It is also just as common for the Smart Meter to be the least of their problems...as was true in our case as well. Smart meter guards are readily available and two different kinds tested very well on our electric meter. A guard can block and/or absorb a large portion of the RF emitting from the device. It doesn't eliminate everything, instead it leaves just enough signal strength for the meter to send its information to the power company successfully, therefore it will cause no problems with the utility company either.

Wall outlets

Whenever possible, try to keep the head away from a wall with an active outlet, and don't run extension cords or power cords beneath beds. We own our own EMR testing meters so that we can test our exposure to EMF, RF, DE and magnetic frequencies. This is a simple, yet effective way to empower yourself with solutions based on real time readings. Consider investing in the tools to equip yourself with the power of knowledge.

WiFi

The most effective solution to WiFi exposure is to have your house wired with grounded, shielded Cat 6 ethernet cable. Shielded and grounded wires prevent EMR fields. We plan to hardwire our home eventually, but in the meantime we use power line adapters which transmit the internet via the electrical wiring in the house. It's brilliant really! As long as the electrical system is updated and efficient, this is a great (and inexpensive) workaround, preventing you from having to have the whole house wired with ethernet cables.

You connect one power line adapter to a router (which must have the ability to turn off the WiFi scanning) via an ethernet cable (grounded, shielded Cat 6 ethernet cords), and the adapter is plugged into a wall outlet. Then you have one or more additional adapters that you can plug into any wall outlet throughout the house, which you will then connect to your computer via ethernet cable. Interestingly, the service is often faster using this method. Since this means you are going to be using a wired connection, I discovered a fabulous little gadget called "Cord Pro" which allows you to wind up the cord so you can unwind as little or as much as you need. It keeps things tidy so you aren't tripping over wires all over the house. In our house, there could be four of us using devices at one time, which can get unsightly and confusing, even with our Cord Pros. I can't even imagine if we had fully unraveled cords all over the floor around us!

Another dilemma we had to solve was regarding our TV. Obviously if you have satellite, there won't be any interference with the removal of WiFi, but if you have a smart TV, you just connect it to a powerline adapter via the ethernet cable, problem solved....BUT, be aware that for many televisions you can't turn off the WiFi component. If you truly want zero WiFi scanning from your TV, you will need to either buy a smart TV that allows you to turn off the WiFi completely, like Sony, or you can have the WiFi component professionally removed from the TV. Devices like Roku, Apple TV, and the stick must be considered too, WiFi can't be turned off on them, they would have to be fully unplugged. You can unplug devices that are not in use and at minimum, you would want to at least turn off your router completely at night. Sleep is supposed to be a time of healing and regeneration. There is a bit of a trade off involved in this solution to WiFi, so it is also important to know that while using powerline adapters you will increase dirty electricity in your wiring. This can also be tested with a meter and filtration devices reduce the dirty electricity, if needed. There is yet another trade off. Reducing dirty electricity with filters increases magnetic fields. As overwhelming as this can all feel, keep in mind that all of these fields can be tested for and corrected by partnering with a Building Biologist who comes to your home for an assessment and then helps you devise a plan to mitigate sources of exposure. My thought process on the trade off is that WiFi is in the air and can't be avoided, while electrical and magnetic fields can be physically avoided, because they tend to dissipate with distance (unless there is a wiring problem in the home which could actually increase magnetic fields immensely). We uncovered a pretty significant faulty wiring event in our kitchen, of all places. We spend a good portion of our time in meal preparation. The result of the faulting wiring was a significantly elevated magnetic field around our island encompassing almost the entire walkable space in our kitchen.

Note - Don't use powerline adapters or filtration devices within close proximity to your headboard or anywhere you will spend a lot of time physically. When in doubt, put money towards a metering device or a professional who can test for you.

Unplugging

A simple and highly effective solution to ambient EMR exposures throughout the house (sourced from inside the house) is to unplug. When you aren't using devices such as chargers, toasters, lamps, TVs, blenders, radios, etc…unplug them!! Leaving them plugged in, even when they are off, results in elevated EMR in the room and DE in the house by accumulation.

Imagine the cord is like a hose with a sprayer nozzle on the end. When the nozzle is turned off, the water is still pressurized inside the hose, just waiting to be released by the sprayer. Your wired appliances and devices are exactly the same way. The electricity is sitting in those wires like a dam of electricity just waiting to be released when you turn them on. This creates cumulative electrical currents throughout the room (and the wires) which add to your body voltage which can be measured with a body voltage meter.

If unplugging the devices in the room isn't enough to obtain ideal sleep levels, experiment with turning off breakers at the electrical panel, but be sure to use a body voltage meter to identify which breaker combinations offer the safest results, because turning off breakers causes cancellation effects that can actually increase body voltage in other rooms, in certain situations. There are various levels of switches that can help make this process more streamlined, you can even have a cut off switch installed at the panel which is controlled by a remote from the living area. See the website link under "EMR reducing supplies" in the website listings at the end of this book for these types of products.

There is just too much we don't know about the potential risks associated with EMR exposures. We are participating in a giant human experiment while developing dependency on a technology that is proving to be a serious health hazard.

---

1. M Havas and D. Stetzer, *Graham/Stetzer Filters Improve Power Quality in Homes and Schools, Reduce Blood Sugar Levels in Diabetics, Multiple Sclerosis Symptoms, and Headaches,* Environmental & Resource Studies, Trent University, Peterborough, ON, K9J 7B8, CANADA, Stetzer Electric Inc., http://www.electricalpollution.com/documents/Havas&Stetzer_revised.pdf

ENVIRONMENTAL PROBIOTICS

This is an up and coming industry that I consider absolutely brilliant! We use probiotics to balance the bacteria in our guts, because it works by mimicking nature's ability to balance the microbial terrain, and now we can use probiotics in our environment to control pathogenic microbes in the air in the same fashion! When we were navigating the mold remediation process in our home, I had done quite a bit of research aimed at balancing the environment. Back then, all of these trendy boutique companies didn't exist yet, but I did find a few mom and pop suppliers of environmental probiotics. I spent a small fortune to have them ship me a gallon of their product so that I could bring the microbial balance in our house back to a healthy place post-remediation. Thankfully, there are companies popping up all over now.

The newer products are also more user-friendly, offering handy spray bottles and time-released atomizers for hands-free maintenance. When you spray these little guys around your house, they literally gobble up all the bad guys (microbes). It helps to create microbial harmony in your living space. This is a phenomenal way to deal with fungus, bacteria and viruses in the environment. It is a safe alternative to killing everything with chemicals and because the probiotic essentially eats the pathogen, it leaves no dead bugs behind in it's wake! It's the dead bugs that cause many allergies because they leave mycotoxins behind.

If you have ever had a mold problem in your home, or if someone in the family is sick, this sort of product will make a huge impact in your life! The applications are endless: you can spray your furniture regularly to keep it free of dust mites and microbes, spray the soil of your plants (or pour it into their water), put a few sprays into your garbage can after putting food in it to prevent odor from bad bacteria, spray your sponges, dishwashers, showers and tubs, they are great for pet beds and toys and even to spray right onto your pets, you can use it for musty front loading washing machines, for cleaning off new furniture (or used) that enters your home for the first time, spray your damp bath towels down, your door knobs, handles and light switches, and for those of you who have guests from moldy houses visit for the weekend, you can even spray them and their belongings down! We also like to periodically clean our phones (cell phones and house phones) as well as any remote controls with it. The probiotics will continue to clean the surfaces you spray it on for days! I don't travel anywhere without my probiotic spray. Hotels are host to all kinds of travel buggies.

In a demonstration I watched, the probiotic spray was compared with Lysol wipes. A bacterial count was taken from two cell phones, one had a count of 120 while the other had a count of over 1500. The cell phone with the count of over 1500 was sprayed with the probiotic spray then wiped off. The other phone was wiped with Lysol, allowed to sit for a moment, then also wiped off. The initial results showed the Lysol to be more effective, leaving zero colonies of bacteria behind on the cell phone, while the probiotic spray still had a count of 5 colonies (down from 1500 remember). But wait for it...an hour later, the untouched phones were tested again. The Lysol-treated cell phone was back up to 104 colonies of bacteria (almost the same as the original count) and the cell phone that was cleaned with the probiotic spray had only **one** colony of bacteria! It continues to work for days!

For heavier applications, there are environmental probiotic products that can be used with inexpensive foggers, while new plug-in distribution methods are offering additional application methods. One company even offers a unit that is installed into the HVAC ductwork. This option is appealing since it eliminates germs inside the air ducts in your house, which typically requires a professional company to even reach them. It then blasts the probiotic out into the rest of the house on a set schedule. No hand sprayer necessary! Since newer fiberboard heat ducts can't be cleaned, this is a wonderful application for houses with fiberboard ductwork. Some environmental probiotic companies make hand sanitizers, home sprays, dental appliance and toothbrush cleaners, soaps, shower gels, pet-specific products and yet another has developed facial and hair products. We love spraying our hands before going out into public or using restrooms and then again afterwards. Just make sure to verify that the other ingredients are safe for your family.

For anyone dealing with mold, this is something to seriously consider. For families dealing with PANDAS/PANS you will have to experiment cautiously, because there are many strains of bacteria (even good strains) that will trigger a flare. We have used soil based organisms (SBOs) as our internal probiotic and most of these environmental probiotics are also made form soil based organisms. So, if you are able to take the SBOs internally, it's safe to assume that you should be ok with the home sprays too. I have found that we react to some brands, but have done well with others that don't cause any reactions. Sometimes I've noticed that even with our preferred brands, if we go too long without using them, we will have some die off in our sinuses associated with breathing in the spray, but wiping surfaces with a rag that is sprayed with the probiotic, rather than spraying it into the air, reduces this minor reaction.

ESSENTIAL OILS

Oh, do we love our essential oils! In fact, I have my diffuser running in the room, as I write this! I know more than a handful of people whose children have been recovered largely in part with essential oils. Essential oils are concentrated, liquid plant extracts used for aromatic and wellness purposes. They are called "essential" because they contain the essence of a plant. Essential oils come from a variety of plant sources, including flowers, grasses, fruits, roots, trees, and leaves. Like homeopathy, they will raise your vibration, increasing your vital force while triggering healing in your body according to their uniquely individual strengths. They can be used in a diffuser, topically, and in some rare cases, internally, but please consult a professional before ingesting any essential oils. I love creating custom combinations to be used in a warm bath.

The business of essential oils is a big industry, and growing with popularity, so you will likely know or be able to find someone selling them quite easily. Find companies that align with your quality standards and mission. It is important to know that there is no agency that oversees the quality of essential oils in the United States, so there is no specific standard that qualifies as "therapeutic grade." This term is a trademarked term. There is, however, a standard that should be upheld by any company you choose to purchase from. Do your due diligence in checking into whoever you choose to use.

Very interesting little side note - Behind the belly button lies something known as the Pechoti gland. *"Through blood vessels, ligaments, nerves, and fascia, the belly button is also connected to the organs in our abdomen, our brains, and ultimately, to the rest of our bodies."*[1]

Applying oil (even everyday oils like coconut oil, olive oil, almond oil, neem oil, mustard oil, ghee, castor oil or any others with healing potential) via the belly button offers yet another healing twist. In

Ayurvedic text, Nabhi Chikitsa is a specialized treatment of pooling oils into the naval cavity to combat certain disorders.

My boys and I occasionally apply a CBD and Frankincense mixture into our belly buttons. It's another alternative to accessing the blood stream without ingesting the oil.

————————————————

1. "The Button that Connects Body and Brain," (Jun 2016),Â https://www.ilchi.com/the- button-that-connects-body-and-brain/

FLAME RETARDANT

Mattresses, upholstered furniture, carpeting, carpet padding, insulations, curtains, car seats, loose pajamas and more…what do these things have in common? Oh wait, I gave it away with the heading, didn't I? Flame retardant chemicals have been linked to serious health risks, including infertility, birth defects, neuro-developmental delays, reduced IQ, behavioral problems, hormone disruptions, and cancer. According to the Environmental Working Group, who independently studies chemicals found in household items:

> *"Fire retardants are commonly added to furniture containing polyurethane foam, including couches and upholstered chairs, futons and carpet padding. They also turn up in children's products such as car seats, changing table pads, portable crib mattresses, nap mats and nursing pillows. Some TVs, remotes, cell phones and other electronics, as well as building materials, also contain chemical retardants, but these sources are much more difficult to avoid. Foam products made before 2005 may be the most hazardous. Older foam items commonly contain PBDEs, highly toxic fire retardants that were taken off the U.S. market. But scientists are finding that newer substitutes such as TDCIPP may be just as harmful, so EWG recommends buying products made without fire retardants whenever possible."*

From an article on Dr. Mercola's website about fire retardants in the home,

> *"Moreover, the chemicals do not remain inertly bonded within the foam or upholstery. They escape in the form of dust, making their way into everything from babies' mouths to breast milk and water supplies. One recent study found that every dust sample collected from American homes contained Tris phosphate(TDCIPP) and triphenyl phosphate (TPHP). Ninety-one percent of urine samples from the residents also contained metabolites of Tris phosphate, and 83 percent had metabolites of TPHP. This echoes other tests, which have shown that an estimated 90*

percent of Americans have flame-retardant chemicals in their bodies, and many have six or more types in their system. American mothers have levels of flame retardants in their breast milk that are about two orders of magnitude greater than in European countries where these chemicals are not permitted, and children have been found to have levels of flame retardants that are as much as five times higher than their mother's. Needless to say, bioaccumulation can have serious health consequences over the course of a lifetime, although health problems may not be readily attributable to day-to-day chemical exposure."

According to Linda S. Birnbaum, director of the National Institute of Environmental Health Sciences,

"Some of the effects that we're seeing are effects on the developing nervous system. We're seeing effects on the developing reproductive system. In a population of children that have been exposed to the flame retardants, those children have lower I.Q., more difficulty in learning."

Considering the increased rates of learning disabilities in our nation's children, it would be worth investing in healthier options and yes, they do sometimes cost more, but so does extended health care. Your family's health is worth the investment.

We have personally seen sky high levels of antimony (heavy metal and fire retardant ingredient) reduce to normal after consciously avoiding pajamas with fire retardants and replacing our boys' mattresses with organic, chemical free mattresses. It was only a matter of months before their hair tests (Doctor's Data, the Toxic and Essential Elements test) were re-done and they were in the normal range. To find pajamas without fire retardant, make sure they are the tight-fitting pajamas. Anything loose will contain fire retardant chemicals like antimony.

GEMMOTHERAPY

Gemmotherapy is an easy to learn, supportive modality that would compliment literally any other modality! But don't let the simplicity of this healing gem (pun intended) cause you to put it on the back burner, because this plant stem cell therapy is a powerhouse! The healing potential from Gemmotherapy alone is nothing short of miraculous, especially for those struggling with proper elimination. It has the potential to set your central nervous system back on track! Combined with homeopathy, I have personally seen it result in astonishing changes, and fast.

Gemmotherapy is aimed specifically at providing support for the adrenal glands, the lymphatic and circulatory systems, and for the bowels and kidneys. Supporting these organs leads to improved immune response, cleaner cells and a reduction in inflammation. Gemmotherapy supports proper elimination which aids in the elimination of toxins, slowing down accumulation. It's safe to say that everyone with either an acute or chronic illness could benefit from Gemmotherapy.

HOMEOPATHIC HOME KIT AND SELF-CARE BOOK

I would highly recommend purchasing a simple homeopathic home kit, especially if there are babies, children, pregnant women in the house. Homeopathy is even wonderful for pets and plants!! It is great for emergencies and can be paired with a self-help guide for using homeopathy in acute situations around the home. It is not a substitute for real emergencies which require the assistance of a trained professional, but homeopathy can be used in combination with any other modality of healing without interference.

Starting out with a home kit will give you the encouragement to take charge of your family's health, and even if you use a homeopathic practitioner, having the kit provides you with the arsenal you will need for acute dosing at the direction of your homeopath. I discovered the incredible value of our home kit each time we had a middle of the night acute illness! There are many reputable companies who carry home kits. I started out with a 50-remedy kit from Washington Homeopathic which is available on Amazon.

I chose to become a homeopath, because of the sheer magic we experienced with homeopathy. I highly recommend having a professional homeopath to slowly and gently promote long-term, permanent healing. Modalities that are natural, don't necessarily heal if they are used in a way that causes suppression of symptoms. An herb, while created by nature, can be potent and it can suppress, so while I appreciate the modulating benefits of many herbs, I have learned the hard way that they can also be harsh, especially when used inappropriately. Homeopathy doesn't suppress symptoms, it encourages the body to seek out and produce healing of the root cause. The difference is that the BODY does the healing, not the remedy. The body takes it's signals from the remedy and it enriches the vital force. It is however, very important to work with a homeopath who aligns with your ideals on healing. Please interview them and follow your intuition on who feels right for you.

LAWN CARE (AND THE NO-SHOE RULE)

Imagine this, an 8-month-old is crawling around on the floor, sitting, playing, then crawling again and of course she is also putting her hands and her toys in her mouth. Her dad walks in from outside, he walks right up to her and lifts her high into the air for a big hug and kiss, then sets her back down and walks across the room while she returns to playing on the floor. Can you envision his footpath, across the room and right up to her, then past her? Now imagine all the foot traffic that comes in and out of the house every single day, all day, from the family, kids running in and out, friends visiting and even Fido. Can you see the swirling array of foot paths all over the house now? Think about what might be on this little girl's hands if she plays on the floor daily.

I am an advocate for allowing the natural defense mechanism to be triggered by microbes, it's how we develop immunity from a young age, but what I am not a fan of, is the chemicals in the mix. We do not develop immunity to chemicals! If you (or your neighbors) are using any form of chemicals (especially Roundup) in your lawn care, not only does this contribute to the toxicity of this planet, but it contributes to the array of toxins being tracked into (and all over) the house.

Whether or not you have an infant, these chemicals get caught up in dust particles around the house and then as you walk, they are stirred up into the air where you are going to inhale and ingest them. Yum! So you can kill two birds with one stone by eliminating the chemical lawn care. Sure, you can take off your shoes at the door, and I highly recommend you do that anyway, because it's not just lawn chemicals that are tracking into your house from the soles of shoes, but Fido can't remove his shoes and we all know that there is the occasional, "Oh, I just need to grab...and it's upstairs, in the other room...it'll just be one second" moments. If you rely solely (pun intended) on taking off your shoes at the door, then you must also keep your shoes at the entrance to the house or carry them with you to and from the door so you don't walk through the house in them.

So, now that you are going to stop using chemicals on your lawn (because you are, right?) you want to know what to do about your lawn. How do you keep your lawn looking spiffy? You have to keep up with the Jones', right? Or do you? That is up to you, but if you are concerned about your lawn and really don't want to feed the bees with dandelion fields from your yard just yet, you can find companies that specialize in organic and safe lawn care. Just know that organic does not necessarily mean safe. The two are often assumed as being interchangeable, but with lawn care, that is't the case.

We've used NaturaLawns of America for years and LOVE the results, I truly mean, love. Our lawn is like a carpet! Their plans are customizable so you can truly design the plan that fits your style and needs. There are also many online sources of DIY lawn care with organic and natural product recommendations. The best way to avoid weeds, is quite similar to our internal terrain…weed and seed, and balance the nutrients. The more beneficial plant growth you can encourage, the less weeds you will experience. Are you seeing the trend?

Oh and to go back to the no-shoe house rule. A study conducted by the University of Arizona found large numbers of bacteria both on the bottom and inside of shoes: averaging 421,000 units of bacteria on the outside of the shoe and 2,887 on the inside.

"The common occurrence (96 percent) of coliform and E. coli bacteria on the outside of the shoes indicates frequent contact with fecal material, which most likely originates from floors in public restrooms or contact with animal fecal material outdoors," said Gerba. "Our study also indicated that bacteria can be tracked by shoes over a long distance into

your home or personal space after the shoes were contaminated with bacteria."[1]

Transfer of bacteria from the shoes to uncontaminated tiles ranged from 90% to 99% according to the study. Some of the bacteria found on the shoes included: Escherichia coli, known to cause intestinal and urinary tract infections, meningitis and diarrheal disease; Klebsiella pneumonia, a common source for wound and bloodstream infections as well as pneumonia; and Serratia ficaria, a rare cause of infections in the respiratory tract and wounds. Need I say more? I found another good use for that environmental probiotic!

———————————————————————

1. https://www.ciriscience.org/a_96-Study-Reveals-High-Bacteria-Levels-on-Footwear

LIGHTBULBS

It is mind-boggling to me that health advocates are recommending (and using) CFL (Compact Fluorescent Light) bulbs which contain and emit mercury in the name of energy conservation. When did saving energy become more important than our health? Just because it saves energy, doesn't mean it's safe. The manufacturing process alone is harming countless people and our environment. Once the bulbs are produced and circulated, they are continuing to contribute to the mercury in our air, soil and water, especially when they are broken (and I say "when," not if, because eventually they WILL end up in a disposal system somewhere and eventually a landfill, where they WILL be broken, emitting the stored mercury into the air).

Although it sounds like a minuscule amount – 4 to 5 milligrams – there is enough mercury in just one fluorescent light bulb to contaminate 6,000 gallons of water. Imagine what that will do to our already elevating toxins in the oceans. They are contributing to pollution with one of the most dangerous heavy metals on the planet, a potent, developmental neurotoxin that damages the brain, liver, kidneys and central nervous system.

It has also recently been discovered that CFLs, as well as LEDs, emit dirty electricity which is known to trigger health problems. According to The Alliance for Natural Health,

> "CFL bulbs contains other cancer-causing chemicals as well. German scientists found that several different chemicals and toxins were released when CFLs are turned on, including naphthalene (which has been linked to cancer in animals) and styrene (which has been declared "a likely human carcinogen"). A sort of electrical smog develops around these lamps, which could be dangerous."

I don't know, it seems like a no-brainer to me, these are best to be avoided. Many are just blindly trusting the environmentalists who say this is eco-friendly. It's a conundrum and it's going to bite us in the behinds. In our home, we've continued to use incandescent and halogen bulbs.

If you already own some of these dreaded bulbs and you need to properly dispose of them (although, I'm not convinced there is any way to "properly" dispose of mercury) you can find a recycling center near you here - https://www.epa.gov/cfl/recycling-and-disposal-cfls#whererecycle

If you break a mercury-containing lightbulb in your home, the following are the clean-up guidelines suggested by the EPA:

- People and pets should immediately leave the room.
- Open a window and/or door and Air out the room for 5 to 10 minutes.
- Turn off the central forced air heating/air-conditioning system.
- Thoroughly collect broken glass and visible powder using wet cloths. Never use vacuum cleaners or brooms.
- Put all debris and cleanup materials in a sealable container and put outdoors in a trash container or protected area until materials can be disposed of properly. Do not leaving bulb fragments or cleanup materials indoors.
- If practical, continue to air out the room where the bulb was broken and leave the heating/air conditioning system shut off for several hours.[1]

---

1. http://www.epa.gov/cfl/cflcleanup.html

PERSONAL CARE PRODUCTS

Our skin is the largest organ of our body and it is highly effective at absorbing whatever you apply to it (with some exceptions).

In our house, if we can't eat the ingredients (or at least recognize and pronounce them), it doesn't touch our skin. This is another effective and inexpensive way to reduce your toxin load considerably, because everything that goes on your skin, has the potential to end up IN your body and these are products typically being used on a daily basis.

This would include anything that touches you in any way: toothpaste, mouthwash, deodorant, soap, shampoo, conditioner, shaving cream, lotion, sunblock, body wash, bubble bath, make-up, feminine care products like tampons and pads, etc.

I always start my research for commercial personal care products with the Environmental Working Group, because every ingredient has been tested and rated, making it easy to find the top products in your category. Homemade options are also available on Etsy and you will often find great recipes online to make your own custom products. As with anything we eat, we prefer organic GFCFSF (gluten-free, casein-free and soy-free) products, whenever available.

SILVER HYDROSOL/COLLOIDAL SILVER

Silver is a natural antiseptic, so it must be used with caution, but in place of pharmaceuticals, it is a great solution to have on hand for hard-to-beat infections like strep throat, bronchitis, pneumonia, MRSA, all kinds of wounds and more. Unlike antibiotics though, it doesn't create resistant strains of microbes.

Don't over use it, after all, it IS a metal and an antiseptic (natural antibiotic) so it will influence the gut flora, but if you would like a first line of defense for hard to treat bugs, this is one of the big guns in our house. When in doubt, call your doctor.

I've read that silver hydrosol would be THE go-to product in the event of bio-warfare, although that will depend heavily on the microbe involved. I hope to never see the day when there is a massive attack of this kind, but I like knowing I have this wonderful natural antibiotic-substitute on my side, in the event of something that catastrophic!

SUPPLEMENTATION

Restricted diets, expressed gene mutations in the methylation pathways, and microbial overgrowth predispose us to potential nutritional deficiencies requiring supplementation, but be aware that it is possible to go overboard. There are many protocols that take supplementation to the extreme. Where available, pure or food-based supplementation is always a better choice, because synthetic forms of anything can accumulate and become toxic. There is also the possibility that synthetic nutrients and additives aren't even properly utilized by the body since they may be recognized as toxins which tend to become sequestered as part of the defense mechanism of the body. I've also recently been made aware of elevated levels of glyphosate in supplement capsules, which generates concern about the source of the capsules.

When you begin supplementation, it is important to treat each new supplement like a new food being introduced to an infant. Introduce only one at a time and watch for reactions/ changes before adding anything else. I would even go as far as to introduce a small portion of the suggested dose amount and work your way up to the visibly improved dose. Keep everything else the same during this transition. Changing other things during this process can confuse things.

Supplementation should be re-evaluated regularly and in some cases, testing may be essential with certain nutrients, especially fat soluble supplements. We have used a variety of supplements and through trial and error, have discovered that for us, less is more. Below is just a core list of baseline supplements to consider, we rotate other things in and out, as needed.

B-12

Most of our kids (and probably even most of us parents, since our kids get it from us) have a deficiency in B-12 due to methylation breakdown. Having the MTHFR gene mutation puts you at greater risk of being deficient, but knowing which other mutations exist in the methylation pathways is critical prior to randomly supplementing with methylated B-12, because it can be problematic for those with COMT or MAO mutations due to the way some neurotransmitters are broken down. In our case, we we are over-methylaters and see a multitude of unsavory behaviors associated with MB-12 (methyl B-12) and gene testing confirmed my suspicions about why. We carry an active MAO gene mutation.

Hydroxycobalamin which is slower-release and longer acting, is more widely accepted and is considered safe for all types of genetics. It is the only form we tolerate. So if MB-12 results in a worsening of symptoms or B-12 levels don't improve with supplementation, consider hydroxycobalamin which easily converts to methyl B-12 in the body, so the job still gets done!

B-Vitamins

Digestive disorders prevent the body from properly absorbing B vitamins, making this a common deficiency seen in Autism and PANDAS/PANS. B vitamins help your body break down food and convert it to energy.

If you experience an intolerance to B vitamins resulting in a worsening of symptoms, there could be a few factors to consider:

- Gene expression may be triggered for those who have a tendency to over-methylate (see B-12 above)
- Magnesium may need to be increased. Antibiotics deplete vitamins B1, B2, B6, B12, folate, calcium, magnesium, potassium and vitamin K (which is quite telling since beneficial bacteria also produce these exact nutrients).
- Micro-doses of supplemental lithium enhances folate and B-12 transport into cells.

Cell salts - see detailed explanation under "Nutrition."

Chanca Piedra/Phyllanthus Fraternus or Stone Breaker

Phyllanthus Fraternus is an Arjuvedic herb that has been used as a supportive therapy for gallstones, kidney stones, malaria, diabetes and hypoglycemia, acute and chronic pain, bacterial and viral infections, high blood pressure, high cholesterol and hepatitis B. Its affinity for many organs makes it a powerhouse herb for supporting not only detoxification, but the effects oxalates have on the body, as well. I had been using this herb on and off for oxalate accumulation, as needed, when I came across research that suggested that this herb also has the unique ability to protect the brain from the damage of EMF exposure. This quickly became part of our daily routine. I began adding it to our oil and lemon blend which supports the liver and gallbladder.

Cilantro

We use cilantro to kick up the natural elimination process. It is helpful in the detoxification process by binding with toxic metals and excreting them via urine and feces, but because it has an uncanny ability to mobilize more toxins than it can carry out of the body, we pair it with chlorella (see more about chlorella in "nutrition" and "toxins"). We take chlorella thirty minutes prior to cilantro tincture and then follow-up with a good binder an hour or two later, to be sure everything that was mobilized exits the body. It is also a known superfood, because of its extensive source of vitamins and minerals. This combination nicely supports detoxification from sauna and IonCleanse foot bath use.

Equisetum tincture

Also known as horsetail, this herb contains high levels of silica which, among other things, is known for pulling aluminum out of the body. It also relieves bed-wetting by supporting the kidneys, it nourishes the bones and is considered a treatment for osteoporosis, and strengthens connective tissue. Since horsetail contains an enzyme that can deplete vitamin B1, you will want to be aware of potential thiamine deficiency which can cause weakness, fatigue, weight loss, irregular heart rate and emotional disturbances like night terrors, panic attacks, depression, irritability, headaches, nausea and abdominal discomfort. People with Chronic Fatigue Syndrome do very well on higher doses of thiamine suggesting there is a direct connection between energy loss and thiamine deficiency. Good dietary sources of thiamine are: pork, beef, poultry, organ meats, legumes, brewer's yeast, nuts and black strap molasses.

Iodine and its co-nutrients

We have either used Lugol's iodine or chlorella. There is also a detailed explanation of chlorella under "Nutrition." Chlorella contains small amounts of iodine naturally, so if you require larger amounts, supplementing with Lugol's is ideal. All iodine supplementation should be paired with important co-nutrients such as selenium and vitamin C, at minimum. I would recommend looking into Dr. David Brownstein's work regarding iodine deficiency and supplementation. See a detailed explanation of iodine under "Nutrition."

Magnesium

Magnesium and B6 is recommended for ADHD and ASD because of it's calming effect on the central nervous system. Magnesium should be split up throughout the day into smaller doses for better absorption.

There are multiple forms of magnesium, each with it's own strength and weakness.

This breakdown from the Magnesium Advocacy Group details the purpose of each form of magnesium:

- Chloride - Detoxing, metabolism, kidney function
- Citrate - not recommended, as it interferes with Ceruloplasmin and can cause iron dysregulation and health issues
- Glycinate - Relaxing, good absorption rate, leaky gut, nerve pain

- Malate - Energizing, fibromyalgia, muscle pain
- Oxide - Good in small doses throughout the day
- Sulfate - Small oral doses, best in bath
- Taurate and Orotate - Cardiovascular health
- Threonate - Brain injuries, PTSD, depression, neurological conditions, anxiety
- Mag water - One of the co-factors, improves absorption

Omega 3 fatty acids

Supplementation is required, because omega 3 fatty acids can only be obtained through dietary sources. The compounding problem of an increasingly toxic ocean and sea life prevents us from sourcing enough seafood from our diet to fulfill our body's requirement of omegas. Testing of fish from various parts of the world, even some of the most pristine locations, are now resulting in findings of psychotropic drugs, antibiotics, nuclear radioactive chemicals from the fallout of Fukushima and of course, mercury. The sheer volume of fish necessary to supply enough omega 3s would certainly cause mercury toxicity, at minimum.

We have used fish oil in the past, but with continued toxicity concerns over anything from the ocean, we have decided to forego ocean-sourced anything. Fish oil is the concentrated fat from various parts of the fish, and toxins store in fat cells, so you should be concerned with purity, at minimum, if you are going to use fish oil for your omegas. My boys didn't really do well on fish oil anyway so we use a plant-based supplement.

Camelina oil which is wild flax, is more stable than conventional flax, meaning it is not prone to rancidity, because of a unique antioxidant complex. The seed oil contains an exceptional (up to 45%) amount of omega-3 fatty acids. It helps that it tastes better than fish oil and conventional flax too! It has a grassy flavor, and is even tolerated by my salicylate sensitive little guy. We all do great on it and I've noticed more stable and mellow behavior from the boys when we are consistent with this supplement. For Gavin, I mix his

Chanca Piedra into his morning oil. Grayson and I take it with a spoon of olive oil, lemon and Chanca Piedra.

Another form of Omegas to consider would be algae from fresh water farms. Just be sure you research the source and that they can provide you with third party testing.

Probiotics

According to the National Human Genome Research Institute, the human body is host to approximately ten times as many non-human microbial cells to human cells. This equates to 100-150 times more genes than there are in the human genome, 3 million versus 23,000! Genes determine function, they send messages out for function. Numerous scientists argue that the combined DNA of our probiotic residents are more important to our survival than our own DNA! The messages from the gut are telling the brain how much hormone and neurotransmitter to make, etc. The fact that for every one message going from the brain to the gut, there are _nine_ going from the gut to the brain demonstrates the importance of the makeup of our resident bacteria.

The gut controls everything and we now know that gut health influences Autism and PANDAS/PANS. Since most of us has been on an antibiotic at least once in our lifetime, the gravity of the consequence of nuking our immune system is dire. Research suggests that antibiotics can disrupt the gut for six months and that there is a collective intelligence in the microbiome of a family unit [22], where the microbiome of other family members matches the persons' who was on the antibiotic.

The moment our beneficial bacteria are drastically reduced like this, opportunistic bacteria, fungi, and parasites rush in to fill the ecological void. Considering 90% of what we are as humans comes from bacteria, we unequivocally must protect our resident microbial colonies. And since so far no study has been able to show that supplemented strains remain in the body for more than two to four weeks, protecting our native microbiome must be a top priority in our lives and the lives of our vulnerable children. These same studies do demonstrate that supplemented probiotics assist our native probiotics strains though. The probiotic strains pass on information to our native strains that they will retain for as long as they survive, as well as forming a defense for our native probiotics, allowing our probiotics to proliferate.

So it's obvious that no health plan (no person) is complete without regular, if not daily inoculation with probiotics. Probiotics inhibit pathogenic bacteria, reduce intestinal permeability, support liver function, reduce incidence and duration of illnesses, increase immune response, improve gastrointestinal problems, decrease inflammation, reduce allergic response, mediate fever, aid in detoxification, produce vitamins, enzymes, fatty acids, peptides, neurotransmitters and even reduce mycotoxins from exposure to mold, among many other crucial tasks. Considering 70-80% of our immune system is in our gut, it's safe to say that gut health is paramount to overall health.[1]

Probiotics are ideally acquired through the regular intake of fermented foods. You are more likely to be familiar with probiotics in yogurt, sauerkraut and pickles, but there are other fantastic dietary options you may be less familiar with like: kimchi, kefir, natto, kombucha, tempeh and Lassi. The problem with commercially fermented foods is the questionable level of beneficial bacteria actually present in the product by the time it reaches your home. Most commercial products also have some form of preservative which may or may not influence the living organisms.

Fermenting your own food is more likely to result in optimal bacteria levels. In some countries, eating fermented foods with every meal is commonplace. In the USA, fewer and fewer people are exposed to sufficient amounts of good bacteria, due to a disinterest in culturing foods at home. Sadly, it is also becoming more and more common for chronically ill people to react to the histamine produced by the wild bacteria in fermented foods, as a result of the imbalance of the microbiome, thereby reducing exposure to these essential bacteria even further. It can become a vicious cycle.

Adding insult to injury, we are regularly surrounded by gut-damaging foods and chemicals on a daily basis. It was even recently disclosed on the Microbiome Masterclass that emotional health influences gut health. This is a two-way street. We are seeing an influx of data related to the gut-brain connection. With 50% of our neurotransmitters in our gut and 90% of our serotonin produced here, it goes without saying that gut health deserves to be a consideration in ALL health conditions, both mental and physical.

But did you know that probiotics also _produce_ nutrients? According to research pulled together by Case Adams, PhD in his book "Probiotics, Protection Against Infection", probiotics are responsible for producing vitamins B1, B2, B3, B5, B6, B7, B9, B12, co- enzyme Q10, K2, K7 and vitamin A, to name a few. Unlike dietary vitamins which are mainly absorbed in the proximal part of the small intestine, the uptake of microbial nutrients mainly occurs in the colon, which contributes to overall systemic vitamin levels. But probiotics don't just produce vitamins, they're also critical to nutrient absorption![2]

- They increase the bioavailability of copper, calcium, magnesium, iron, manganese, potassium, and zinc
- They break down proteins and fats for digestibility
- They break down and process carbohydrates and sugars
- They increase digestibility of milk and phytonutrients
- They bind to and reduce blood levels of cholesterol

There is no coincidence that the imbalance in the gut of those with chronic illness is directly related to these deficiencies and also explains why synthetic supplementation often isn't sufficient to address them. We absolutely need the beneficial gut bacteria present in order for the proper assimilation of our nutrients to take place!

And it's important to note here, that not all good bacteria or probiotics colonize in the gut.

They don't all hang around permanently once they enter our
systems. Many of the benefits we see from probiotics are produced
by strains that are actually transient, meaning they pass through
rather than taking up residence. This is another good reason to
ingest probiotics daily. Cultures around the world rely on fermented
foods at every meal and we can begin to see why when we learn
more about the role probiotics play in our health.

Our choice probiotic is **flourish by entegro**, because it is a living,
liquid probiotic, meaning it is 100% viable, whereas powdered and
encapsulated versions are 2-70% viable, upon reconstitution.
According to entegro, all probiotics start out as a liquid; they have
to be grown as a liquid. To encapsulate the probiotics, they have to
be centrifuged to remove most of the liquid (and as a result, the
food source and the beneficial metabolites are lost as well). After
being centrifuged, the paste is then freeze-dried into a powder. This
powder can then be placed into capsules or mixed with other ingredients. In this process, the bacterial strains are typically grown as
single strains and combined only after having undergone centrifuga-
tion and freeze-drying; they did not grow together in community.
Flourish retains the natural growing state, never centrifuging or
freeze-drying. Also, all eleven strains are grown together in a
commensal environment. By remaining in the natural liquid state,
their food source and all the good metabolites that the beneficial
bacteria have produced are retained. Also, growing communally
ensures that the bacteria can thrive together, benefiting one
another.

To demonstrate the effectiveness flourish can offer, just one table-
spoon of flourish is equivalent 4-5 bottles of kombucha! Since it is a
liquid product, starting out with lower doses couldn't be easier!
Some people need to start out at drop-doses, because of it's potency
and the resulting die off, so I recommend buying an amber glass

dropper bottle to dose from. Note - flourish contains a strain of strep.

Probiotics have held a strategic role in our recovery. It was absolutely a turning point in health for all of us, because it began the essential task of repairing the damage in our guts. As a health coach and homeopath, this product has also been pivotal for many of my clients. To learn more about the product go to entegrohealth.-com/jessica. If you would like to join my Facebook group, search for "let's flourish! Jessica for entegro."

Pyroluria

In the most simple terms, pyrrole disorder is when your body creates too many pyrrole molecules. Pyrrole molecules bind with zinc and B6. A healthy person excretes pyrroles in their urine on a daily basis with no problem. Someone with pyrrole disorder excretes too many pyrroles and in turn too much zinc and B6. This is problematic because zinc and B6 are vital for your digestive system, immune function, cognition function, and emotional balance.[3]

> "Children in a pyroluric state are volatile, angry, and tend to cry easily. They are often calm one moment and angry the next for no apparent reason. They have a great deal of inner tension, and often manifest their symptoms with impulsive unfiltered behaviours. If you are working with a child who goes into frequent rages and is inconsolable and continually acting out, this can be a sign of pyrrole disorder. Children with pyroluria may have sensory issues. They are often sensitive to tags on clothes and certain fabrics against their skin. These children need down time to calm down after an up-cycle of bad behaviour. They may prefer to be alone or find themselves isolated and alone because others prefer not to be with them. These children often experience a worsening of symptoms during growth spurts. One possible but not definitive sign of pyroluria in children is multiple white spots on the fingernails."[4]

With proper supplementation, many people experience relief within several days of treatment. A more substantial recovery could take up to 6 months, with greater improvement occurring gradually over 3-12 months.

Take the self-test below. If you are B6 and zinc deficient, you will easily identify with some of the following symptoms.

CHECK YES TO ANY OF THE FOLLOWING QUESTIONS:

- When you were young, did you sunburn easily?
- Do you have fair or pale skin?
- Do you have a reduced amount of head hair, eyebrows, or eyelashes, or do you have prematurely gray hair?
- Do you have poor dream recall or nightmares?
- Are you becoming more of a loner as you age? Do you avoid outside stress because it upsets your emotional balance?
- Have you been anxious, fearful, or felt a lot of inner tension since childhood but mostly hide these inner feelings from others?
- Is it hard to clearly recall past events and people in your life?
- Do you have bouts of depression and/or nervous exhaustion?
- Do you have cluster headaches?
- Are your eyes sensitive to sunlight?
- Do you belong to an all-girl family, or have look-alike sisters?
- Do you get frequent colds or infections, or unexplained chills or fevers?
- Do you dislike eating protein? Have you ever been a vegetarian?
- Did you reach puberty later than normal?
- Are there white spots/flecks on your fingernails, or do you have opaquely or paper-thin nails?

- Are you prone to acne, eczema, or psoriasis?
- Do you prefer the company of one or two close friends rather than a gathering of friends?
- Do you have stretch marks on your skin?
- Have you noticed a sweet smell (fruity odor) to your breath or sweat when ill or stressed?
- Do you have or did you have, before braces crowded upper front teeth?
- Do you prefer not to eat breakfast, or even experience light nausea in the morning?
- Does your face sometimes look swollen while under a lot of stress?
- Do you have a poor appetite, or a poor sense of smell or taste?
- Do you have any upper abdominal, splenic pain? As a child, did you get a "stitch" in your side when you ran?
- Do you tend to focus internally (on yourself) rather than on the external world?
- Do you frequently experience fatigue?
- Do you feel uncomfortable with strangers?
- Do your knees crack or ache?
- Do you overreact to tranquilizers, barbiturates, alcohol, or other drugs-mat is, does a little produce a powerful response?
- Does it bother you to be seated in a restaurant in the middle of the room?
- Are you anemic?
- Do you have cold hands and/or feet?
- Are you easily upset (internally) by criticism?
- Do you have a tendency toward morning constipation?
- Do you have tingling sensations or muscle spasms in your legs or arms?
- Do changes in your routine (traveling, new situations) provoke stress?
- Do you tend to become dependent on one person whom you build your life around?

Score_____ If you scored 15 or more, it is possible you are suffering from zinc and B6 deficiency.

This questionnaire was originally developed by author, researcher, and clinician Carl Pfeiffer M.D., Ph.D a pioneer in the field of biochemistry.

Selenium

Selenium has been reported to increase immunity, has positive antiviral effects, is essential to fertility, defends against free radical damage and inflammation and even reduces the risk of cancer and thyroid diseases. As mentioned above, when taking any form of iodine, it is important to also get enough selenium. Selenium is taken in very small quantities and can even be obtained through the diet.

Foods high in selenium are brazil nuts, liver, sunflower seeds and eggs. We have had to use a yeast-free form of selenium rather than food, because of the dietary restrictions that prevent my kids from eating nuts, eggs and yeast. We do occasionally use a liver supplement though. Be aware that too much selenium can cause: muscular weakness and fatigue, nausea, vomiting, nervousness, loss of hair and a bad odor on the fingernails.

Vitamin C

Also an essential co-nutrient of iodine, Vitamin C is responsible for a multitude of functions within the body and is required for tissue growth and repair, as well as detoxification. It also blocks the damage created by free radicals, thereby reducing cancer risks. Not getting enough can cause easy bruising, gingivitis, bleeding gums, dry hair, dry skin, decreased wound healing rates, nosebleeds and a decreased ability to ward of infections.

Vitamin C is water soluble, meaning it is not stored by the body when used in excess, however, for families with the tendency to accumulate oxalates, supplemental vitamin C must be used with caution, at very very low doses, if at all. We prefer to eat a lot of fruit, leafy green vegetables, bell peppers, broccoli and some blueberries and strawberries (which are moderate in oxalates and require moderation). On the rare occasion that we get sick, I will sometimes give VERY small quantities of lyposomal vitamin C to temporarily and quickly boost immunity. Gavin naturally gravitates to camel milk when he is sick, drinking it almost exclusively until he is better. Camel's milk has about three times as much vitamin C as Cow's milk.[5]

Vitamins D3 and K2

Since we don't use fish oil and we live in the Northern Hemisphere, another vital supplement in our household is vitamin D3 and while it is not the purest supplement, due to processing, I believe the benefits far outweigh the risks, especially since it is also very unlikely to cause toxicity issues when paired properly with vitamin K2.

Without proper K2 levels, colecalciferol (D3) is known to cause hypercalcemia (an abnormally high level of calcium in the body) so supplementation of the two together is necessary for proper absorption and transport of calcium. We never dose vitamin D3 without K2.

1. M.Y. Soon and S.S. Yoon, *Disruption of the Gut Ecosystem by Antibiotics*, Yonsei MedJ. 2018 Jan 1; 59(1): 4-12. Published online 2017 Nov 29. doi: 10.3349/ymj.2018.59.1.4, PMCID: PMC5725362, PMID: 29214770
2. Case Adams, P.hD, *Probiotics: Protection Against Infection*, Logical Books (2012)
3. http://www.mensahmedical.com/pyroluria-pyrrole-disorder/
4. C. Talty, M. Dahlitz, Pyrrole Disorder for Therapists, Oct 1, 2013, DOI: 10.12744/tnpt(3)058-066, https://www.thescienceofpsychotherapy.com/pyrrole-disorder-for-therapists/
5. Z. Farah, R. Rettenmaier and D. Atkins, *Vitamin Content of Camel Milk*, Internat. J. Vit. Nutr. Res. 62 (1992) 30-33, Received for publication September 5, 1991, https://camelmilkforhealth.com/publications/ journal_for_vitamin_and_nutrition_research_62_1994_30.pdf

Recommended reading

THERE IS no better way to learn than to surround yourself with good literature by those who have been successful in the subject you want to know more about! I can't say it enough, if you are on a journey to learn more, read, read and read some more. My recommendations are certainly not all inclusive, but they do serve as some of the best books in their genre so as you scan the lists below, trust your intuition on what jumps out at you first. Always keep a notebook handy for those important tidbits that will lead you to the next chapter of your quest for knowledge.

A NEW EARTH BY ECKART TOLLE

Eckhart Tolle's books are nothing short of transformational. We have so much to learn from exposing and confronting our ego, which subconsciously controls our reactions. We hold the power to liberate ourselves from suffering and Tolle has just the right words to get us there. Just be sure to take your time reading his books, they require time to digest the lessons you will learn. With his bestselling spiritual guide *The Power of Now*, Eckhart Tolle inspired millions of readers to discover the freedom and joy of a life lived "in the now." In *A New Earth*, Tolle expands on these powerful ideas to show how transcending our ego- based state of consciousness is not only essential to personal happiness, but also the key to ending conflict and suffering throughout the world. Tolle describes how our attachment to the ego creates the dysfunction that leads to anger, jealousy, and unhappiness, and shows readers how to awaken to a new state of consciousness and follow the path to a truly fulfilling existence. I found the pain of Autism and PANDAS to be triggering throughout recovery, and learning techniques for remaining present halted and prevented a lot of self-induced trauma.

· · ·

BUDDHISM FOR MOTHERS OF SCHOOLCHILDREN BY SARAH NAPTHALI

You certainly don't have to be Buddhist to appreciate the gentle, compassionate techniques offered in this lovely book. Everyone who wants to guide their children with more patience will glean something from Sarah's teachings. This book explores those teachings through many scenarios, including managing the stress of numerous deadlines, coping with routine and repetition, answering children's tricky questions about how the world works, fitting in with other parents, managing our fears and expectations for our children, and dealing with difficult behaviors in both children and adults. Raising high needs children can elevate stress levels while isolating families so I found her profoundly calm approach to be incredibly inspiring.

She also suggests ways to share Buddhist teachings with children so they maintain a connection to their own inner wisdom rather than reacting to peers and the media. At a time when there is so much "noise" in our daily life, there is something quite soothing about the tools Buddhism can teach us to rely on.

CAMEL CRAZY - A QUEST FOR MIRACLES IN THE MYSTERIOUS WORLD OF CAMELS

This inspiring book was written by a friend who was bravely acquiring camel milk from overseas years before I even set my eyes on it, or her, but it wasn't until she came across my Facebook group, *"Healing with Camel Milk,"* that she felt safe enough with her consistent American supplier to begin sharing her story and research with the world. You see, there was a time when us parents held camel milk very close, out of fear that the dairy industry or the government would prevent access.

A talented author and passionate mother, Christina delivers the perfect balance of experience, humor and information in Camel Crazy. This is her beautifully colorful journey with worldly camel culture and the resulting recovery her son experienced from Autism. While access to camel milk for Christina was riddled with a variety of roadblocks, she was equally gifted with the magical and wondrous global influences that could only be bestowed by these same events. You will get lost in mysterious worlds with her, as you cheer her on for being brave enough to trek the world for this unique passion. Once you've experienced the powerful healing capacity of camel milk yourself, you will quickly come to understand what it means to be "Camel Crazy."

DIRTY GENES BY DR. BEN LYNCH

This book focuses on the genetic expression of a handful of mutated genes in the methylation cycle, which is critical information when used wisely. Educating yourself on the way our genetics can be triggered and how to influence the expression of these genes is part of the huge and complicated world of disease. It is fairly new science that uncovered the truth that the expression of certain gene mutations will trigger specific illnesses. Dr. Lynch does a nice job of balancing these understandings with not going overboard and blaming everything on genetics. He offers a step by step method of detection and management of the genes causing symptoms.

Here is a fun set of statistics found in this book: Bacterial cells in your body outnumber your human cells by 10 to 1 and bacterial genes outnumber your human genes by 150 to 1. Furthermore *we* don't digest fiber, only our gut bacteria do. They ferment it as they feed on it, producing acids and other biochemicals that are vital to a number of different human functions, from digestion to the regulation of thought, cravings and moods. Think about that for a moment, our gut bacteria determines our moods and regulation of thought. With the crap food most people eat, is there any wonder why so many people are chronically crabby, impatient, forgetful and experience brain fog? I would like to thank to Dr. Ben Lynch for confirming my research on this, and for providing well balanced insight into our genetic evolution.

GEMMOTHERAPY FOR EVERYONE - AN INTRODUCTION TO ACUTE CARE BY LAUREN HUBELE

I trained with Lauren Hubele and love her systematic approach to Gemmotherapy. This little book enables you to get familiar with the acute potential of Gemmotherapy. It is quite simple to use acutely, but if your problem stems from chronic elimination issues, it would be a good idea to hire a professional of Gemmotherapy to experience deeper treatment.

Her company, Vital Extract, also sells acute care kits which are an ideal way to introduce yourself (or an expecting mother) to the incredible world of Gemmotherapy. Do it, you won't regret it!

HEALING THE NEW CHILDHOOD EPIDEMICS BY DR. KENNETH BOCK

All I can say about this book is if you have a child with Autism, PANDAS/PANS, allergies, ADHD or asthma, get this book! Get it. *BUT, please understand that I do NOT agree with his suggested form of chelation and use of metal "challenges."* These can be dangerous to partake in, because they use unnaturally high levels of chelators which mobilize a LOT of metals and at the end of the half-life of the chelator, the metals that were in the process of being escorted out of the body, are dropped and become free to redistribute. There are safer ways to detox and many other forms of detoxification remove more than just heavy metals, while chelation moves metals, and metals only. Also, PANDAS/PANS is not specifically discussed in this book, but the causes and treatments are all related. His explanation of why our kids are sick and how these disorders are all related is an education not to be missed, if you are on this train with me.

HOMEOPATHIC SELF-CARE: THE QUICK & EASY GUIDE FOR THE WHOLE FAMILY BY ROBERT ULLMAN

If you are interested in using homeopathy for your family, buy yourself a simple home kit in the 30C potency and a self-care book like this one. It will guide you step by step through the process of identifying a handful of remedies which can then be tried according to personal needs, acutely.

· · ·

How to End the Autism Epidemic by JB Handley

The conundrum of vaccine safety awareness lies in the fact that it requires putting all of the pertinent pieces together by reading a slew of science surrounding multiple topics. The average person would have no clue which studies, or even which topics, will paint the true and accurate picture of vaccine safety issues. It takes enormous manpower, time and knowledge to put it all together and unfortunately most families don't have the time or inclination to make that happen. Until now though, this is exactly what many Autism parents have been doing all. by. themselves. and this is the message they are trying to spread to those around them.

In "How to End the Autism Epidemic", journalist J.B. Handley and co-founder of Generation Rescue, publishes all of the studies and research that he tirelessly pulled together during his plight with his own son's Autism. He has compiled this data in an easy to read (and understand) format, enabling access to this information in one place. It may even serve as a jumping off point to dig further into the thorough research he provides, putting it all right at your fingertips. And although his book aims squarely at vaccines, it's easy to extrapolate facts supporting other potential triggers for regressive and congenital Autism. There is more than enough information provided to highlight the mechanisms involved in Autism, as it relates to environmental factors at large.

Never before have I seen such a thorough compilation of the research coupled with the very details needed to fuse the science with the outcome. It would be nearly impossible to read this book and come away with anything less than certainty that vaccine safety needs more attention.

If you would like to educate loved-ones, new and expecting parents, care-givers, teachers, doctors, local political influencers or anyone else who believes the "science is settled", this book should be on your gift list immediately!

Iodine, Why you need it, Why you can't live without it by Dr. David Brownstein

Thyroid conditions are on the rise. I can't even count how many people I know with a thyroid condition and they range in age from children and young adults to the elderly. Learn what you need to know about the role of iodine in your diet and how a deficiency begins the process of thyroid dysfunction. But the thyroid isn't the only organ system effected by a deficiency in iodine. The reproductive system depends on sufficient iodine saturation in the body, as well. Deficiency during pregnancy can lead to cretinism, a lowered IQ and if severe enough, infant mortality. Iodine supplementation requires co- nutrients, therefore, I would not recommend supplementation without education first.

Natural Healing with Cell Salts by Skye Weintraub, ND
This is simply an easy-to-use repertoire with a complete list of cell salts and ailments.

Outsmarting Autism, Updated and Expanded: Build Healthy Foundations for Communication, Socialization, and Behavior at all Ages by Patricia S. Lemer
This book came out after I was already well on our way to recovery, so I haven't had the pleasure of reading her book yet, but I have met Patricia personally and she is one very dedicated and well-versed researcher on the subject of recovery. Her approach resonates with me and incorporates multifactorial causes supporting her "Total Load Theory" which explains that developmental delays are caused not by one single factor, but by an overload of environmental stressors on genetically vulnerable individuals. This book addresses Autism identification, treatment, and prevention from pre-conception through adulthood. She describes more than 50 practical approaches with proven efficacy, including lifestyle modification, dietary considerations, and boosting the immune system. Wouldn't it be nice to see more focus on prevention? Kudos to Patricia for bringing prevention to the forefront.

. . .

Reset Your Child's Brain by Victoria L. Dunckley, MD: A Four Week Plan to End Meltdowns, Raise Grades and Boost Social Skills

Increasing numbers of parents grapple with children who are acting out without obvious reason. Revved up and irritable, many of these children are diagnosed with ADHD, bipolar illness, Autism, or other disorders but don't respond well to treatment. They are then medicated, often with poor results and unwanted side effects. Based on emerging scientific research and extensive clinical experience, integrative child psychiatrist Dr. Victoria Dunckley has pioneered a four-week program to treat the frequent underlying cause, Electronic Screen Syndrome (ESS). Dr. Dunckley has found that everyday use of interactive screen devices — such as computers, video games, smartphones, and tablets — can easily overstimulate a child's nervous system, triggering a variety of stubborn symptoms. In contrast, she's discovered that a strict electronic fast improves mood, focus, sleep, and behavior, regardless of the child's diagnosis.

Sara Books 1, 2 and 3 by Esther and Jerry Hicks

Everyone on this planet should read these books, adults and children alike! Let Sara and Solomon take you on a journey to learning the truth about happiness and appreciation. Law of Attraction is generated by developing the habits taught in this wonderful story. You won't be able to put these books down! My own kids couldn't wait to read them with me every day, in fact, they made comments like, "This book makes me so happy" and "I love Sara, can we read more today?"

Sensational Meditation for Children by Sarah Wood Valley

Do you want your children to learn and appreciate meditation, but don't know where to start? That is no easy task for the average person, because children don't naturally sit still for very long. Meditation for children absolutely has to be fun if you want them to enjoy it and eventually rely on it as a tool in their self-help toolbox. This book offers 14 different fun, guided meditations for you to experiment with, which will help you encourage your child(ren) to experience the wonders of meditation. You may even find yourself using a few of them regularly. I did!

THE AWAKENED FAMILY: HOW TO RAISE EMPOWERED, RESILIENT AND CONSCIOUS CHILDREN BY SHEFALI TSABARY, PH.D.

This is an absolute favorite of mine. This book had me hooked from the very first page. It opened my eyes to the subliminal conditioning we receive growing up, and made me consciously aware of ways to minimize this effect in our children. This book armed me with skills that transformed my parenting and inadvertently healed some of my own parenting fears. Every page was full of profound material, every one!

THE IMPOSSIBLE CURE BY AMY LANSKY

This was the first book I read about homeopathy and I would still consider it one of the most important books I've read. My homeopathic trajectory began here. Amy Lanky does a wonderful job of balancing memoir with education. For anyone who wants to learn more about homeopathy while discovering the hope it can offer, this is the book for you. It's a must read for anyone considering homeopathy.

THE BIOLOGY OF BELIEF BY DR. BRUCE LIPTON

As was mentioned earlier, this book was a game-changer for me. Once I realized the importance of our environment (physically and emotionally) and how it impacts us right down to the smallest atoms in our body, I felt held to the task of becoming more conscientious of my actions and thoughts. Learning that genes don't cause disease, beliefs do, also encouraged me to teach my children more about the various tools they can pull from to address stress in their lives.

. . .

THE POWER OF NOW BY ECKHART TOLLE

One of the best self-help books I've ever read. The act of staying present takes practice. Eckhart Tolle can weave anything into such identifiable and real terms that it not only makes sense, it becomes easier to incorporate into every day life. In the first chapter, Tolle introduces readers to enlightenment and its natural enemy, the mind. He awakens readers to their role as a creator of pain and shows them how to have a pain-free identity by living fully in the present.

THE THINKING MOMS' REVOLUTION: AUTISM BEYOND THE SPECTRUM: INSPIRING TRUE STORIES FROM PARENTS FIGHTING TO RESCUE THEIR CHILDREN

If you are looking for hope and inspiration from the trenches, this book will deliver. It is a collection of real, raw stories which will touch every emotion in you at one point or another throughout the book. Join these families as they suck you into their world and share their plights with you, me and anyone else who is looking for the light at the end of the rainbow. Twenty-three moms and one brave dad make up The Thinking Moms' Revolution. Their group stretches from Montana to Malaysia to Montreal. I have the pleasure of knowing many of these unique parents and their stories. This book will shed a much needed light on the hope of recovery.

While parenting children with disabilities, they came together on Facebook to collaborate about bio-medical and dietary interventions, as well as doctors and researchers developing cutting edge treatments. In the process they became a tight-knit family dedicated to helping their children lose their diagnoses. Out of this collaboration they have created something far more substantial. Suspecting that the roots of their children's Autism, ADHD, Asthma, Sensory Processing Disorder and food allergies may be found in the overuse of antibiotics, preventative medical care, environmental toxins and processed food, they began a mission to turn it around!

Each chapter is written by a different TMR member sharing how they found each other, what they have learned along their journey, and why the support of close friends, also parenting kids with special needs, is so important. In this book you will read about their individual experiences, and learn how their determination and friendships have become a daily motivation for parents worldwide.

In follow-up, TMR has also produced **Evolution of a Revolution, Thinking Grandparents** and keep an eye out for their upcoming puberty book. Proceeds go to the TMR grant program where parents can apply for funding to help with the cost of therapies for their children.

$\mathcal{W}$ ebsites

SINCE WEBSITES CAN CHANGE RAPIDLY, this list may become outdated over time, but even if the particular website listed isn't available, it may spark research into others like it.

ASK HEALTHY JESS

This is my website. It is a collection of the information I've gathered throughout the years of our journey. I have been heavily researching and experimenting with how to achieve true health for over a decade, and I am now able bring all of this together here for you.

I developed askhealthyjess.com to offer a mindful solution to the growing options on the internet. It can be overwhelming to navigate a journey to better health when there is so much information at your fingertips. Becoming overwhelmed to the point of paralysis is a real thing! Paralysis is a roadblock to healing (wink).

On Ask Healthy Jess, you will find product recommendations, mold testing information, dietary intervention links, recommended FB groups to assist in your journey, nontoxic product recommendations and more.

The goal with Ask Healthy Jess is to bring all of the pieces of healthy living together in one place, reducing the frustration that comes with the overwhelm of too many choices. The content is likely to change and/or grow regularly so visit often. See you there soon!

ANTENNA AND CELL TOWER SEARCH

Find cell towers and antenna structures within a 4 mile radius of your home. Don't let the "antennas" fool you into thinking they are safer than towers, the only difference is often related to their height, not their output. An antenna can be just as powerful and dangerous as a cell tower.

- Antenna Search - antennasearch.com

BioPure

BioPure is Dr. Klinghardt's supplement brand. His products are recommended throughout the book due to their purity and success track record. Whenever possible, they use organic ingredients and formulas that are free of unnecessary binding agents and fillers. The only chlorella we will use is BioPure's Chlorella Growth Factor capsules. We've reacted negatively to everything else. From their website:

In addition, we use a number of other practices to ensure purity, safety and maximum efficacy:

- Real-time sourcing
- Flash freezing for 100% phytonutrient potency
- Advanced sublimation technology (freeze drying)
- No irradiation or EtO (ethylene oxide)
- GMP- and HACCP-compliant encapsulation facilities

All of our products are diligently tested according to FDA guidelines and certified with a COA (Certificate of Analysis). Many of our vendors run laboratory tests such as DNA certification, Essential Run Tests on pesticides and herbicides, and a mass spectrometry to identify possible adulterants. Our bottlers test for physical qualities such as the color or odor of a raw ingredient and run selective-sample assay tests congruent with batch numbers as an additional safety measure to ensure quality and consistency.

Lastly, a panel of national and European naturopathic and medical physicians runs comparative "double-blind" Energetic

Testing (also known as Autonomic Response Testing) on all of our products. Our test kits are updated regularly and available to the growing number of Health Care Practitioners using this type of prognostic tool to support their treatment plans.

- BioPure - BioPureUS.com

BUILDING BIOLOGY

Create Healthy Homes - Building BiologyTM began over thirty years ago in Germany as "Bau-biologie"TM in response to the decline in health caused by the rapid rise of toxic, improperly constructed buildings in post WWII Europe. The founders of the profession created alternative design and construction practices to reverse this trend. This site was created by Oram Miller, BBEC, EMRS, a certified Building Biology Environmental Consultant and Electromagnetic Radiation Specialist who is based in Los Angeles. His website is full of great tips for creating a healthy home. On this website you will find a host of videos, as well as explanations on various topics related to EMF sources and solutions for mitigation. His website has very detailed educational information.

International Institute for Building-Biology and Ecology - Here you can learn more about how to create a healthy home and locate seminars on subjects including: building physics and building biology, EMFs and air quality. You are also able to search for local certified experts to conduct an assessment of your home. There is a link with a handful of architects and builders, as well as products and stores!

- Create Healthy Homes - CreateHealthyHomes.com
- International Institute for Building Biology and Ecology - hbelc.org

CAMEL MILK AND AUTISM

Christina Adams is an American award-winning writer, journalist, author and speaker. She and her work have been featured by National Public Radio, The Washington Post, The Los Angeles Times, LA Times Magazine, Gulf News, Khaleej Times, Dubai One, GOOD, Open Democracy, OZY, Autism File, Global Advances in Health and Medicine, WebMD and more. Her books, "A Real Boy" and "Camel Crazy" reveal the world of Autism and her son's early intervention. Her series "Autism and Beyond" airs on Autism Live at www.autism-live.com. An expert on Autism and camel milk, she advises families and scientists from many countries and enjoys connecting with and learning from people from all cultures.

- Christina Adams Author- ChristinaAdamsAuthor.com

CHILDREN'S HEALTH DEFENSE

Robert F. Kennedy, Jr. as the founder of the Children's Health Defense, lawyer, researcher and advocate, aims to end the epidemic of children's chronic health conditions. He is an environmentalist and humanitarian who walks the talk shedding light on issues influencing the declining health of our children.

- Children's Health Defense - ChildrensHealthDefense.org

DIETARY SUPPORT

It's no secret that dietary interventions are hailed as some of the most important changes that can be made in the lives of those with chronic illness. Dietary changes can also be some of the most intimidating tasks on this journey. Below are a few resources to help you get started, but don't limit yourself to these links. There are so many dietary resources available on the internet, these are just a few of the tried and true that I value for clarity and accuracy.

FAILSAFE DIET

The failsafe diet is designed to treat intolerances or sensitivities to specific chemicals in foods. The diet is not designed to treat allergies. Reactions to food chemicals are pharmacological and dose-related rather than immune-system related, but they cause a number of symptoms that appear to be allergy-like. It should be considered, at minimum, if any of the following diagnosis are present:

- Pervasive Developmental Disorders (PDD)
- Asperger's Syndrome
- Attention Deficit Disorder (ADD)
- Attention Deficit Hyperactivity Disorder (ADHD), hyperactivity, nervous energy, fidgety
- Autism, co-morbid Autism spectrum disorders
- Dyscalculia, dyslexia
- Dyspraxia
- Epilepsy, seizures
- Head banging
- Learning difficulties
- Obsessive Compulsive Disorder (OCD)
- Oppositional Defiance Disorder (ODD)
- Picky eating
- Sensory Integration Dysfunction (SID), Sensory Processing Disorder (SPD)
- Speech delay
- Speech disorders, speech impediments, stuttering
- Tic disorders, Tourette's Syndrome

For a complete list of symptoms and guides on which foods are safe, go to the website.

- Failsafe Diet - FailsafeDiet.com

Low Histamine

For support in reducing histamine foods or balancing low histamine eating with anti-inflammatory foods, Yasmina offers numerous recipes, workshops and cookbooks.

- Low Histamine Chef - HealingHistamine.com

Low Oxalate Diet (LOD)

For some reason, the information online for the LOD is some of the most inconsistent I've seen. Many websites are very inaccurate in regards to which foods are low oxalate and which aren't. Mislabeling a food's oxalate content potential can be highly deleterious to the reduction of oxalate accumulation in the body. We once tried a type of green bean for a summer (only on rotation, not even very often, maybe once a week) and it resulted in weeks of oxalate dumping when we recognized that we were actually increasing oxalates too much. It can be disheartening and deflating to encounter speed bumps like this while trying to do your best to improve the health of a loved one. So please be careful with the oxalate information on random websites.

I'd actually recommend the Facebook group called "Trying Low Oxalates" as a first resource, because researcher and group founder, Susan Owens, who has dedicated over 25 years to testing and studying how oxalates effect health, has the most up to date oxalate-containing food spreadsheet available. Her research is the most current and pulls together data from multiple trusted sources.

The challenge with oxalates is that the same type of food grown in two different environments can have completely different oxalate contents. So when it comes to oxalate accumulation and dumping, it's best to know the symptoms and trust your gut (no pun intended there) when it comes to which foods feel best.

Websites to help you navigate the LOD (low oxalate diet)

- Facebook group - https://www.facebook.com/groups/TryingLowOxalates/
- OxVox - OxVox.com
- LowOxalateDiet - LowOxalate.info

TACA - FOR THE GFCFSF DIET

This is an invaluable tool when you are embarking on starting the GFCFSF (gluten-free, casein-free, soy-free) diet. TACA stands for *The Autism Community in Action*, but these dietary interventions benefit anyone with chronic illness. This website offers an introduction to the diet, provides step-by-step guidance and offers resources like how to read labels, where you will find hidden ingredients, how to start the diet with an older child (or any older human for that matter), as well as great facts on what these proteins are and why you should avoid them. There are printable shopping lists, ingredient substitutions, a recipe database, money saving tips, how to handle school situations and so much more. TACA also has local chapters that may be available to you. Getting to know others in the same boat as you is empowering.

- TACA - TACAnow.org

DR. MERCOLA

Find news, products and articles by Dr. Mercola, a pioneer in sharing the latest up and coming health information and resources. From his website, *"Dr. Mercola envisions a future where visits to clinics and hospitals are few and far between, and reliance on drugs, surgery, and expensive medical procedures are greatly reduced because of natural health solutions and lifestyle changes."* For an overall glimpse into maintaining a healthy lifestyle, Dr. Mercola's website is a good contribution to variety in knowledge.

- Dr. Mercola - DrMercola.com

EMF/EMR REDUCING SUPPLIES

I would consider this the EMR reducing superstore of the internet. You will find everything you could think of to help reduce EMR exposures in and around your home. Here you will find meters, shielding products, books, educational videos, low EMF appliances and even raw materials to make your own products.

- Less EMF - LessEMF.com

ENVIRONMENTAL HEALTH TRUST

Stay up to date on the science proving that EMF can be biologically hazardous. Since the Telecommunications Act of 1996 (Section 704) states that no health or environmental concern can interfere with the placement of telecom equipment such as cell towers and antenna, it is even more important that we are seeking out this information for ourselves. Environmental Health Trust is the only nonprofit in the world today that both carries out high-level critical research on controllable environmental health hazards and works directly with local communities, teachers, parents and students as well as policy makers to understand and mitigate these hazards through research, education and advocacy. They develop multi-media science-based tools to educate individuals, health professionals and communities about public health threats, as well as identify, evaluate and mitigate risks of cellphone and other forms of microwave radiation by:

- Promoting public understanding of the complex science underlying avoidable environmental health hazards by working with teachers, parents and students to create entertaining, engaging hands-on multi-media

educational tools based on state-of-the-art information that rely on peer-to-peer mentoring
- Conducting cutting-edge research with our world-class collaborators intended to promote new or improved safety standards for cell phones and other microwave radiation sending or receiving devices
- Publishing articles in peer reviewed journals about avoidable environmental health hazards, and
- Working with local, state and national decision-makers and scientists to develop and promote constructive policy changes that rely on our research and extensive input from relevant experts.

- Environmental Health Trust - EHTrust.org

Furniture

Reputable eco-friendly and non-toxic upholstery is very hard to come by, but there are a few companies doing it right. I'm sure many more will surface in the years to come, but for now, these are a few recommendations:

Cisco Brothers

They have an amazing upholstery line called "Inside Green" which is non- toxic on all levels. Their products are made with responsibly harvested woods, organic cotton, latex and wool and their seating support is made with jute and hemp. They are high quality, custom made pieces that don't sacrifice style or comfort. We own two of these couches and will continue to give this company our business in the years to come. They are located on the West Coast in the US, but there are furniture showrooms throughout the US that sell and display their products. We were able to test out a few models at a showroom in an adjacent state. Their styles range from modern to traditional, all with a shabby chic feel.

- Cisco Brothers Inc. - CiscoBrothers.com/inside-green

VIESSO

This is another top of the line furniture manufacturer who doesn't compromise design or comfort in their eco-friendly line of furniture. They have a line of upholstered products made with 100% natural latex, eco wool and organic cotton as well as locally sourced woods, recycled fabrics and reclaimed woods. They advertise the use of low VOC wood finishes, natural linseed oils and waxes and organically grown materials. Their furniture tends to have a more modern flare with mid-century, clean lines.

- Viesso - Viesso.com/eco-friendly.html

ORGANIC AND HEALTHY INC.

This website offers more than just furniture and unfortunately their furniture line is limited, but I am impressed that they have personally researched every item on their website. They have non-toxic products such as mattresses, bedding, furniture, carpeting, water filtration systems, and air purifiers that they have researched for use in their own home to protect their own family, in hopes of helping others create a cleaner indoor environment. This will be a continually expanding product line-up.

- Organic and Healthy - OrganicandHealthy.com

GEMMOTHERAPY WITH LAUREN HUBELE

The place to go for your Gemmotherapy extracts, as well as training with Lauren Hubele. Lauren's extracts are exclusively produced by Europe's leading production facility for homeopathy and Gemmotherapy.

- Vital Extract - LaurenHubele.com

GLOBAL CONSCIOUSNESS PROJECT

Learn about the project results for various globally recognized events that have taken place over the past two decades. The cumulative data suggests that there is most definitely human collective consciousness at work and that we are more intimately connected than we realize.

- http://noosphere.princeton.edu/youtube.html http:// voices.nationalgeographic.com/2011/09/06/9-11-and-global-consciousness/

GLUTEN-FREE SOCIETY

For everything you want to know about how gluten effects the body! The Gluten-free Society was founded by Dr. Peter Osborne, who has been featured in many health summits as a guest speaker. Often times referred to as "The Gluten Free Warrior", he is one of the most sought after alternative and nutritional experts in the world. His private nutritional practice is centered on helping nutritionally support those with painful chronic degenerative and autoimmune problems using natural methods. He is one of the world's leading authorities on gluten sensitivity, and lectures nationally to both the public as well as doctors on this and many other nutritionally related topics. He is the founder Gluten Free Society, the author of The Gluten Free Health Solution and The Glutenology Health Matrix, a series of digital videos and ebooks designed to help educate the world about gluten. In addition, he is the author of the international best selling book, No Grain No Pain, published by Touchstone (Simon & Schuster). He is also the founder and host of The Autoimmune Revolution – an online educational series featuring more than 40 of the world's leading experts on autoimmune disease.

Goals of The Gluten Free Society:

- Educating the world about the broad reaching nature of gluten on human health and disease.
- Providing easy to use, non-invasive tools to help identify people who are gluten sensitive
- Providing instruction through video, audio, and written tutorials for those embarking on a TRUE gluten free lifestyle.
- Providing healthy resources for those with gluten intolerance/sensitivity.
- Supporting research endeavors revolving around grains, gluten, lectins, and other compounds found in grain that may harm human health.
- Providing an ongoing analysis and commentary of research performed in the field of food sensitivity/intolerance.

- Gluten-free society - GlutenFreeSociety.org

Glyphosate Herbicide and How to Detox It with Dr. Stephanie Seneff

Dr. Stephanie Seneff discusses one of the most important health issues of our time – glyphosate toxicity. It's in many non-organic and even some organic foods, and it's ruining your health, causing Autism, gut dysbiosis, problems detoxing and even cancer. This podcast will have you abandoning non-organic foods forever! But even if you eat organic, the glyphosate is still in the water and sprayed on most recreational parks to kill weeds.

Learn what you can do to protect your health and how glyphosate may be contributing to your fatigue and health issues.

Tune in to hear all about:

- How glyphosate causes chronic fatigue, Autism, dementia, gut dysbiosis, cancer and more
- Glyphosate causes mineral deficiencies and oxalates
- Glyphosates contributes to sulphur sensitivity
- How glyphosate makes vaccines more toxic
- How to detox glyphosate

Dr. Stephanie Seneff is a Senior Research Scientist at MIT's Computer Science and Artificial Intelligence Laboratory in Cambridge, Massachusetts. She has a BS degree from MIT in Biology and a PhD from MIT in electrical engineering and computer science. Her recent interests have focused on the role of toxic chemicals and micronutrient deficiencies in health and disease, with a special emphasis on the pervasive herbicide, Roundup, and the mineral, sulfur. She has authored over two dozen peer-reviewed journal papers over the past few years on these topics.

- How to detox glyphosate - https://myersdetox.com/166-glyphosate-herbicide-and-how-to-detox-it-with-dr-stephanie-seneff/

To hear from Dr. Seneff on synergistic poisoning from aluminum and glyphosate at an Autism One conference, go to this link - https://www.youtube.com/watch?v=a52vAx9HaCI

Homeopathy Research Institute (HRI)
If you are looking for the science behind homeopathy and you

want to see studies, this is the place to start. HRI is an innovative international charity created to address the need for high quality scientific research in homeopathy. The charity was founded by physicist, Dr. Alexander Tournier, who previously worked as an independent researcher for Cancer Research UK, conducting interdisciplinary research at the boundaries between mathematics, physics and biology. Those who use homeopathy religiously have typically experienced something of their own, making them believers in this mystical medicine, but if you haven't had your "wow" moment yet, this site might put homeopathy on your radar.

- HRI - HRI-Research.org

INSTITUTE FOR RESPONSIBLE TECHNOLOGY (IRT)
IRT is a world leader in educating the public and policy makers about the health risks and environmental dangers of GMO foods and crops, empowering consumers to lead an organic lifestyle and shaping the changing marketplace.

- IRT - ResponsibleTechnology.org

LYME DETECTION
This is THE lab to use when you are investigating the potential for Lyme Disease as part of a symptom picture.

- IgeneX Inc. - IgeneX.com

For treatment protocols and tips, I would recommend looking into Dr. Dietrich Klinghardt's work at KlinghardtAcademy.com.

MOLD

Investigation into mold can include testing for DNA fragments of mold spores in the home as well as mycotoxins in the home and body. The benefit to testing for mycotoxins in the body, over the home, is that you will know if you or your child are having problems detoxing mycotoxins from the environment. Since we can encounter mold in so many locations, this is a good start towards identifying health challenges associated with mold exposure. If mycotoxin testing comes back conclusive that there is a mold exposure occurring, the next necessary step would be to test the home.

ERMI or HERTSMI testing is ideal, because it detects mold DNA in your dust. Air sampling is another option, however, it often doesn't accurately represent the molds growing within an environment, because there are certain strains (mold is microscopic typically) that are heavier and only remain in the air for approximately 90 seconds. Ironically, it's the more dangerous molds that fit this category, like Stachybotrys and Chaetomium. It's possible to miss these strains completely since air testing is merely a snapshot in time, catching only what is airborne in that particular moment in time. Some companies suggest using a fan to stir everything up prior to air capture, but why stir up dangerous mold spores for a test that you can simply execute using the dust samples from around the house which will more accurately represent the settled mold spores in the home. It is still possible to miss mold growth that is well hidden and sealed up, but it's a good place to start your investigation into the potential for mold in the home.

The links below can help you source testing information for the home and body.

ERMI/HERTSMI TESTING:

- EnviroBiomics Inc - Envirobiomics.com
- Mycometrics - Mycometrics.com

Mycotoxins testing for the body:

Testing can be done without a doctor, via urine testing that is ordered online through LabTests Plus. It is common for the results of this test to mirror ERMI testing results in the house, although mold exposure can occur at school, office buildings, the library, doctor's offices, gyms...etc.

- LabTests Plus - Great Plains Lab Mycotoxins profile - https://labtestsplus.com/product/mycotox-mycotoxins-profile-gpl/

Surviving Mold

Some of the most in-depth mold research will be found here. Surviving Mold was developed by Dr. Shoemaker who devoted his life to finding the answer to illness caused by biotoxins. On his website you will find several additional resources surrounding conventional testing, treatment recommendations, as well as resources for locating conferences and physicians. There is even an online vision screening tool which has the ability to detect changes resulting from biotin exposure. He has also written a book called Surviving Mold.

- Surviving Mold - SurvivingMold.com

National Vaccine Information Center

The non-profit National Vaccine Information Center (NVIC) is an independent clearinghouse for information on diseases and vaccine science, policy, law and the ethical principle of informed consent. NVIC publishes information about vaccination and health to encourage educated decision-making. NVIC does not make vaccine use recommendations. NVIC supports the availability of all preventive health care options and the legal right for individuals to make informed, voluntary health choices for themselves and their children.

- NVIC - <u>NVIC.org</u>

Non-GMO Shopping guide
Products listed have been verified as compliant with the Non-GMO Project standard.

- Shopping guide - <u>nonGMOshoppingGuide.com</u>

Nourishing Hope
Here you will find information about the various dietary interventions discussed earlier in the book. Because body and brain are connected, nutrition affects everything. Nourishing Hope uses scientifically proven methodologies and nutrition-based strategies that are effective at improving the health, learning, and behavior of those with Autism, ADHD, and other developmental delays.

- Nourishing Hope - <u>NourishingHope.com</u>

PROBIOTICS

Oral probiotics
Flourish probiotic is a liquid probiotic, the most natural state for beneficial probiotics to grow and thrive. Most other probiotic products are capsules or powdered. It has been established that between 2-70% of powdered and encapsulated probiotics are activated when they are rehydrated by the body. That is a far cry from the 100%

viable bacteria in flourish, which contains eleven diverse strains of good gut bacteria, including multiple genera: Lactobacillus, Bifidobacterium, Enterococcus, Bacillus, and Saccharomyces. This diversity makes flourish unique because the majority of other probiotic products contain strains from only one or two genera, but not all four. The inclusion of a Saccharomyces (yeast) amongst the other genera is also unique. Flourish probiotics are fermented in old-world style brewing, allowing these eleven strains of bacteria to grow together as a consortium where they will naturally find balance and diversity.

This probiotic blend is kept in its natural [liquid] state along with its prebiotic culture medium (food source) and its naturally produced organic acids, which help the good bacteria to thrive. This provides nutrition and a robust environment for the good bacteria, further ensuring their success. The prebiotic nutrition also feeds the unique probiotic strains that were already present in your gut. Flourish probiotic blend includes nutrition that supports your own individual microbiome. In addition to prebiotics and organic acids, the culture medium provides nutritious vitamins, minerals, peptides, enzymes, short chain fatty acids and amino acids. Being able to take one dose that covers probiotics, prebiotics, and organic acids provides peace of mind that the supplement will successfully supply noticeable whole health support.

We were so impressed with this probiotic that I decided to become a consultant for the company. You can join my Facebook group for more information at "let's flourish!Jessica for Entegro."

- My website to learn more about the product - entegrohealth.com/jessica

ENVIRONMENTAL PROBIOTICS

Indoor air quality is astonishingly poor according to research. As we engage in the interaction with our environment, we are subject to exposure to whatever is found in the air we breath and the surfaces we encounter regularly. Probiotics are naturally found in the air all around us, we are designed to inhale certain beneficial microbes from our environment, perhaps another reason exposing ourselves to nature provides us with such beneficial outcomes. Taking it a step further, the vibrational frequency of beneficial organisms in nature are naturally higher than the toxins that are increasingly showing up in our air quality. And remember, toxins decimate good bacteria. So, just like our bodies which require daily inoculation with beneficial microbes, so does our environment! Much like our gut terrain, our environment is most effective at eliminating toxins when harmony among microbes is achieved. The best way I know how to accomplish this is to bring the outdoors inside. Environmental probiotics are derived from soil based bacteria responsible for cleaning the air and soil by balancing the outdoor microbiome. When used inside on surfaces that collect dust, the probiotics are able to continue working on the surface for days after cleaning with the solution.

By providing our environment with beneficial microbes, we are naturally reducing the bad guys found in our air, like: mold and fungi, pollen, dust mites, various allergens, viruses, and bacteria to name a few. What better way to clean the air, than to balance it with the microbes designed to eat up these invaders! In soil, this is exactly how balance is achieved. In our guts, this is also how balance is achieved.

Now you can create more environmental balance and harmony by using a product that removes these damaging microbes naturally, by improving air quality and benefiting the inhabitants in the building. Because you are using nature to fight nature, you are also preventing the toxic byproduct of killing mold, mycotoxins. Environmental probiotics effectively prevent biofilm buildup on surfaces, reducing the potential for harmful strains to set up shop

I've tried a number of different products and have settled on the one I like best. Just doing a search for environmental probiotics will bring up a list of selections. The link I am providing is for PureBiotics, a brand we've used for years with success. When we had a mold problem brewing in our beach house, we used a combination of a HiTech Air Reactor and cleaned only with environmental probiotics. HERTSMI testing went from a score of 18 (15 and higher is considered unsafe for occupants with CIRS - chronic inflammatory response syndrome) to a 4 (yes, four) within 4 weeks!! A result of under 11 is considered "Statistically safe for re-entry for those with CIRS," although this should really be considered on an individual basis with the types of molds involved being part of the assessment interpretation.

When we were battling mold in our beach house, and my children and I were reacting severely to the environment, we found these little buggers to be priceless at reducing our reactions to mold. We also used them before, during and after remediation of our primary home. I truly believe that our success in remaining in our extensively remediated home without further reactions is related to how we remediated. We never used products that kill or cover up mold. No matter how hard it was to manage financially, we removed the effected materials and replaced them under proper containment from a reputable mold remediation company. Then we continued to balance the microbial communities inside our home by cleaning and fogging with environmental probiotics.

Our preferred company for these household all-purpose cleaners is PureBiotics by Chrisal. We use their All Purpose Professional Cleaner on everything: our counters, floors, all surfaces, cabinets, appliances, even windows. We spray it into garbage cans, our front loader washing machine, the soil of our plants, and we clean our cell phones, house phones and remote controls with it. We take them to hotels to wipe everything down and we even clean the inside of our cars with it. I haven't met a material that doesn't tolerate this product. I also use their mist for misting upholstery, curtains, bedding, pillows, carpet and anything else that can't be wiped down. My couches are all very light beige linen and none of these products have ever stained them.

- PureBiotics - https://purebioticsusa.com/#a_aid=jgal25

PERSONAL CARE PROBIOTICS

In addition to using probiotics in our home and in our bellies, we use them topically on our bodies as well. We use a body wash and oral rinse for cleaning toothbrushes, retainers and as a mouthwash, and we spray them onto our hands in place of hand sanitizer when we are in public.

- Probiotic Power - http://p2probioticpower.com/#_1_7u

RECYCLING CENTERS FOR MERCURY-CONTAINING LIGHT BULBS

https://www.epa.gov/cfl/recycling-and-disposal-cfls-and-other-bulbs-contain-mercury#whererecycle

SEARCH DR. RUSSELL BLAYLOCK ON YOU TUBE

You will find information about vaccines and immuno-excitotoxicity, microglial cell activity and the fragile balance between glutamates and GABA. I know these subjects may sound foreign to you, but I promise, you want to know what he has to tell you. There is a lot to glean from his expertise on the subject of excitotoxicity, which ultimately kills brain cells.

THE ENVIRONMENTAL WORKING GROUP DATABASE

This is an absolute *must-have* resource to have handy for anything that will go into your home or onto your body. They conduct third-party testing on household and personal care products, plus they are expanding their testing to include other things like tap water and water filters. They provide a ton of insightful information about all things toxic.

- EWG - EWG.org

THE TRUTH ABOUT CANCER

After losing many family members to cancer, Ty Bollinger began the tireless task of interviewing countless doctors, researchers and survivors about healing cancer through alternative methods. Although the focus of TTAC is cancer, much of what is promoted for cancer healing can also be used to heal other chronic illnesses, which tend to be precursors to cancer. Why wait until you or someone you love is faced with a cancer diagnosis to start your research? The subject of prevention is woven throughout his website and docu-series.

- TTAC - TheTruthAboutCancer.com

THE TRUTH ABOUT VACCINES

From the people who brought you TTAC, after seeing connections with vaccinations, Ty Bollinger expanded his reach to include this complex arena, as well. In this 7-episode series, 60 top experts will shed light on the history of vaccines, vaccine risks and safety concerns and a list of options and alternatives.

- TTAV - TheTruthAboutVaccines.com

THINKING MOMS' REVOLUTION

It's a blog, a book (three now), a YouTube Channel, a non-profit organization and they offer eConferences and Webinars. A group of informed and experienced parents joined forces to bring information of all kinds to the community of families with children who have disabilities of all kinds. There is also a link to their IonCleanse study results on their website.

- Thinking Moms' Revolution - ThinkingMomsRevolution.com

Vaxxed, From Coverup to Catastrophe (the documentary)

As I was writing this book, a senior scientist from the CDC came forward and admitted to falsifying data in a 2004 study that showed a link between the MMR and Autism. The study, which happens to be the same study doctors quote when they say "the science has been settled, there is no connection between Autism and vaccination", actually discovered that there was a 340% increase in Autism for a subset of children, if they were vaccinated with the MMR vaccine before 36 months of age. Thompson himself was recorded saying that he felt remorse for the 10 years that these facts were covered up. He even went as far as to seek Whistleblower protection through a specialized lawyer. The movie, Vaxxed, was produced by Del Bigtree, a journalist and producer for "The Doctors." He thoroughly investigated and reported his findings. See my blog entry about this event, along with many links, here: http://yourwhatyoubelieve.blogspot.com/search?q=whistleblower and my review of the movie as well as a copy of a letter William Thompson himself wrote in response to the public outcry (and probably the CDC's way of attempting to cover their behinds: http://yourwhatyoubelieve.blogspot.com/2016/04/vaxxed-from-cover-up-to-catstrophe.html

- The Vaxxed official website - VAXXEDtheMovie.com
- Vaxxed II, The People's Truth - is the sequel about the Vaxxed bus tour - VAXXED2.com

VAXXTER

Vaxxter is a site that promotes alternative health news. It's the ultimate guide to vaccine information and more.

- Vaxxter- Vaxxter.com

WiFi in Schools

This is a link to the paper - Evidence that Electromagnetic Radiation is Genotoxic: The implications for the epidemiology of cancer and cardiac, neurological and reproductive effects by Dr Neil Cherry, Lincoln University, New Zealand, June 2000 http://wifiinschools.com/uploads/3/0/4/2/3042232/neil20cherry20presentation1cancerrf.pdf

More from Dr. Neil Cherry

Links to his published papers and articles http://www.neilcherry.nz/document-downloads.html

OUR SYMPTOMS

*B*elow you will find a list of the symptoms that accrued over the first two years of Grayson's life. It is my opinion that with each vaccination, his symptoms deepened, but it wasn't until his overt reaction at one year of age, that we started to make the connection.

- Significant **sleep disturbance** lasting well over six months and involved me having to go to sleep when he did at 7pm, just so I could enjoy the first 4 consecutive hours of sleep each night. The rest of the night was riddled with waking/crying episodes every 45 minutes all. night. long. for at least 6 months, and even when we got his sleep figured out, he still often woke at least 5 times a night, but at least went back to sleep more easily.
- **Colic**, which in hindsight, we now know was due to the formula he was being fed. Formula is a dairy product and is filled with GMO corn syrup solids, which are harmful to beneficial bacteria and feed bad bacteria.
- **Chronic ear infections**, of course resulting in prescribed antibiotics that harm critical beneficial gut

flora. I later discovered that the antibiotics Grayson was put on encourage the overgrowth of insidious pathogenic microbes in the clostridia family.

- **Chronic rhinitis** was evident from birth until we removed dairy years later. Also an indication of microbial imbalance.
- **Loose stools** which lasted most of his early life. Another indicator of microbiome imbalance.
- **Regression after vaccinations** and with illnesses, eventually leading to a backslide that no longer recovered on it's own.
- **Sensory processing disorder (SPD)** even from very early on like hating dirty hands to the point of severe tantrums and sensory defensiveness resulting in him hating cuddles or hugs, he pushed away from us from BIRTH, no joke. I have a picture of him pushing hard against his father while we were still in the hospital. He arched his back away from me during nursing which was a culmination of sensory and dietary related issues.
- **Auditory functioning disorder**, which was part of the sensory dysfunction, caused him to say "What?" frequently. It would appear like he didn't hear us, but it was more about surrounding sounds that caused confusion in what he was hearing. We had his ears tested and they were fine, although nutritional deficiencies did cause a lot of ear wax to chronically accumulate in his ears.
- **Sound sensitivities** associated with the SPD caused him to scream while squeezing his ears hard or to react physically. One time he punched me in the face for flushing a very loud public toilet when I was crouched down at his level helping him. Another time he literally scaled his father's 6 foot tall body to get away from a nearing motorcycle outside. Fear of sudden loud sounds would set off a cascade of high cortisol responses to everything following the event.

- **Frequent rocking** while sucking his fingers hard enough to cause bleeding.
- **Severe startle reflex** requiring swaddling until infant swaddles no longer even fit him. I had to cut the bottom of them open so that he could still have his arms swaddled tightly for sleep well beyond the typical age of swaddling.
- **Hand flapping** when he was excited and/or upset, and this was one of the first things to resolve when we began treatment.
- **Incessant lining up of cars** which is a form of inappropriate play. He would freak out if anyone interrupted his rows. He lined up rows and rows of cars all over our couches and floors, and we couldn't touch them for fear of an extreme tantrum. This also resolved very early on with treatment. It did return briefly through a healing crisis with homeopathy, which we found very interesting.
- **Overstimulation couldn't be self regulated**. Even from infancy, if he was overstimulated by bright or busy toys, he would become physically agitated and hyper, then he couldn't fall asleep for a nap or at night, and the sleep problem would snowball creating more sleep loss in the days that followed.
- **Transitions were extremely difficult** for him to navigate.
- When his hair was wet, even having just taken a bath, he had a **wet dog smell**, indicating an overgrowth of fungus.
- He experienced a variety of body, vocal and facial **tics** that shifted and changed from time to time. This was one of our first signs of PANDAS.
- **Hypoglycemia** from food sensitivities.
- **Self-limiting to foods** containing gluten and casein due to the opioid-mimicry of the proteins paired with leaky gut.

- Severe, debilitating **OCD** which interfered with his sleep, eating, brushing his teeth and playing. Another PANDAS symptom.
- Daily **aggression and defiance** which evolved into all out **rage** episodes as he aged.
- Extreme **mitochondrial fatigue** - we thought he was just a chill kid and liked his stroller during busy events and long walks. We didn't experience the toddler-walking struggles most parents go through at age two, when their kids want to walk all by themselves everywhere. By five years old, when he was STILL demanding to sit in a stroller and carriages instead of walking (resulting in wild tantrums) we knew something wasn't right. I once tried to force him to keep walking beside me in a grocery store after having JUST arrived, and he laid on the ground and cried, because he physically couldn't go any further. Later, Organic Acid Testing (OAT) would confirm mitochondrial involvement.
- **Wild tantrums** with a hair-pin trigger. It didn't take much to set him off. 0-60! These tantrums were paired with his low threshold for frustration. There was no ability to cope with stress of any kind.
- He had an **unnatural fear of bugs, birds and dogs**, more of a phobia. He couldn't be rationalized with during these phobic episodes. Just the site of a bug, bird or dog would initiate the fight or flight response, causing him to run and hide or go into a panic attack.
- Significantly **bloated belly** which began in infancy. I recall family members talking about his "cute Buddha belly" well beyond chubby baby days. He looked malnourished with thin, low muscle limbs and bloating.
- **Low muscle tone**
- **Slow growth**, so slow that there were periods when he didn't grow for over a year! And this is after having been in the 95% as an infant.

Drawing conclusions about vaccine damage might involve the microbiome. Considering reversal of Autism in our household involved high doses of probiotics and dietary interventions, this is where research should be headed!

The *Microbiome Safety Project* by Keith Bell has highlighted some interesting details about how the condition of our microbiome might be related to vaccine reactions! This could explain why some people react so severely, while others do not.

> *"Our central hypothesis is that gut microbiota have a significant effect on host response to vaccination where a reduced or absent population of commensal flora coupled with an overgrowth of pathogenic strains may become a microbial predisposition to adverse vaccine reaction. This may include reduced or absent protective microbiota such as Bifidobacteria, Lactobacillus and butyrate-producing Clostridia allowing immune dysregulating Bacteroides and Proteobacteria to be overgrown."* [1]

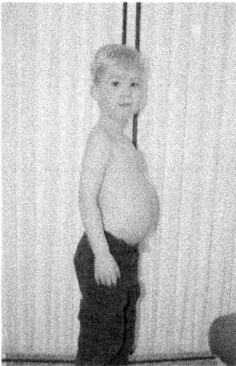

Grayson before gut healing

It's no surprise to those of us who have been in the biomedical trenches for a decade or more, that gut health is directly related to Autism, as well as PANDAS/PANS symptoms! In fact, studies are finally popping up to confirm as much.

With gentle detoxification, dietary intervention and the introduction of soil based probiotics, Grayson's Autism was reversed and PANDAS was put into remission.

Recovery from chronic illness is an intense labor of love. It requires an undying dedication to the person, as well as the belief system that recovery is possible.

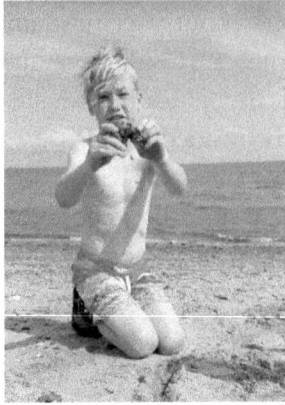

After gut healing

These photos show Grayson before and after gut healing interventions. There is no denying how far his health has come. He continues to gain muscle and endurance as a neurotypical teenager.

───────────

Although Gavin doesn't have Autism, PANDAS or PANS, he has struggled with ODD (oppositional defiance disorder) when his system was imbalanced, and we suspected MCAS (mast cell activation syndrome) which a doctor suggested when he was a toddler. We revisited this condition when he was 11 due to a growing list of sensitivities. We feel grounded in our holistic approaches to health management and using the overflowing bucket mindset from Chapter 13, we've been able to manage his health by controlling triggers.

Below is the list of things we've overcome with Gavin.

- **Low birth weight**
- **Torticollis** shortly after birth (resolved when he started walking, but we also did physical therapy with him regularly).
- **Eczema** in reaction to milk or soy even through MY diet while nursing (removal of the food eliminated his

eczema completely and only food infractions caused it to return).

- **Toenail fungus** - He had one very thick and yellow big toe nail as an infant.
- **Failure to thrive**
- **Febrile seizure** with an illness at 11 months old, resulted in a two day hospital stay and a slew of tests all resulting in nothing out of the ordinary (scariest moment of my life as I watched my child's life appear to slip away from me, in my arms)!
- **Intestinal infections** resulting in a chronic red anal ring.
- **Yeast overgrowth** confirmed via testing.
- **Wet dog smell** when his hair was wet, just like Grayson.
- **Highly sensitive** to touch, used to say "ouch" even when just touching him (this resolved when his gut flora was balanced).
- Frequently **communicated by screaming**.
- **Defiant actions**, especially with his brother. He used physical force even though he never witnessed this sort of behavior in our household.
- He also suffered from **severe bloating** like Grayson, and until we started the low oxalate diet, he had very inconsistent stool consistencies from constipated to loose with a lot of undigested foods (using enzymes eliminated the undigested foods, and the LOD got rid of the stool inconsistencies). Camel milk resolved the undigested food without the need for continuing enzymes.
- **Painful joints and eye pains** (this also resolved with the LOD).
- **Slow speech development** which we didn't quite recognize until camel milk had him suddenly speaking in full sentences, literally immediately!
- Confirmed **parasitic infection - Dientamoeba Fragilis**

- **Significant oxalate and salicylate sensitivities**.
  Oxalate dumping became almost constant until we
  committed to the LOD, we would literally see teaspoons
  of crystals in his urine regularly.
- He **lost two large chunks of his beautiful goldi-
  locks** suddenly one day after starting him on SBOs (soil-
  based organisms). They literally pulled out in my hands,
  the way you would picture hair chunks coming out of a
  chemo patient's scalp. The scalp was smooth, zero hair
  left about the size of two quarters, side-by-side. I
  panicked, we brought him to the doctor for a battery of
  tests, which mostly came back normal, nothing really
  pointing to the cause of the hair loss. His hair did
  eventually regrow in those spots, although the smooth
  spots remained for months without a single sprout of
  hair.
- **Delayed dentition**

Considering the potential connection between gut health and
vaccine reactions, we are so grateful we didn't fully vaccinate Gavin!
This list might have been much worse if we had.

Managing chronic conditions may be a lifelong task, but with a
toolbox full of holistic interventions, one only has to adapt their lifestyle to their needs.

"Genetics loads the gun, environment pulls the trigger" -Dr. Francis Collins

---

1. L. Yuan, P.C. Christina Tsai, K. Bell, *Do gut microbiota mediate adverse vaccine reaction?*
    Virology and Immunology Department of Biomedical Sciences & Pathobi-
    ology Virginia-Maryland College of Veterinary Medicine, USA
    Head of Research & Development, Thryve, USA, Microbiome Vaccine Safety
    Project
    thegutclub.org USA
    https://www.alliedacademies.org/articles/do-gut-microbiota-mediate-
    adverse-vaccine-reaction.pdf?fbclid=IwAR3gnibu1IyAJbuAAgzCfZvlS3SF_eISb-
    F3LSc1d9OP-tFNTrtmMIZMcIOY

INDEX

microbiome 43, 193, 194, 245, 249, 260, 320, 382-384, 417, 418, 427
milk 20, 30, 34–36, 69–71, 80, 155, 180, 216, 235–39, 252, 255, 361, 362, 384, 389, 390, 392, 393, 402, 403
mindfulness 65, 66, 121, 156, 269, 291, 292
mitochondria 38, 39, 88, 194, 260, 427
mold 39, 71, 73, 79, 94, 129, 155, 165–68, 176, 183, 190, 215–19, 311, 317, 318, 321, 355, 357, 383, 401, 413–15, 418, 419
mutation, gene, genetic 203, 215, 377, 378
neurotransmitter 64, 66, 79, 97, 344, 349, 382
nickel 35, 206, 207, 323
O. formigenes 39, 247
obsessive compulsive 17, 73, 404
OCD (obsessive compulsive disorder) 17, 71, 72, 89, 102, 248, 404, 426
ODD (oppositional defiance disorder) 15, 31, 34, 37, 105, 247, 248, 257, 310, 404, 429
omegas, supplemental 177, 381, 382
overgrowth, pathogenic 27, 35, 43, 44, 70, 81, 93, 95, 160, 193, 195, 203, 249, 250, 257, 259, 261, 377
oxalate 38–40, 98, 190, 194, 246, 247, 250, 257, 261, 379, 405, 430
overstimulation 89, 426
PANDAS 15, 64, 69, 71–73, 75, 77–79, 82, 90, 93, 94, 96, 99, 100, 120, 121, 123, 124, 129, 130, 135, 144, 145, 160, 161, 176, 209, 216, 248, 348, 357, 378, 382, 391, 394, 426, 428, 429
parasites 39, 382
PCO (Photocatalytic Oxidation) 165, 166
PDD-NOS 31
PECO (Photo Electrochemical Oxidation) 165, 167
pesticides 100, 175, 201, 207, 245
phone, cell 179, 326, 335, 338, 339, 341–46, 348, 356
Phyllanthus Fraternus (Chanca Piedra, Stone Breaker) 326, 379, 382
plastics 40, 221, 350
potencies, homeopathic 50, 54, 97

www.ingramcontent.com/pod-product-compliance
Lightning Source LLC
Chambersburg PA
CBHW060304030426
42336CB00011B/930